W9-BCC-547

A
GREENHOUSE
FOR THE
MIND

A
GREENHOUSE
FOR THE
MIND

Jacquelyn Seevak Sanders

The University of Chicago Press
Chicago and London

Jacquelyn Seevak Sanders is director of the Sonia Shankman Orthogenic School and senior lecturer in the Department of Education at the University of Chicago. She earned the Ph.D. in education and psychology with a focus on curriculum at the University of California, Los Angeles, and is a licensed psychologist.

The University of Chicago Press, Chicago 60637
The University of Chicago Press, Ltd., London
© 1989 by The University of Chicago
All rights reserved. Published 1989
Printed in the United States of America

98 97 96 95 94 93 92 91 90 89   54321

Library of Congress Cataloging-in-Publication Data

Sanders, Jacquelyn Seevak.
    A greenhouse for the mind / Jacquelyn Seevak Sanders.
    p. cm.
    Includes index.
    ISBN 0-226-73464-1
    1. Child psychiatry. 2. Mentally ill children—Education.
I. Title.
RJ499.S26 1989
618.92'89—dc19   88-23346
                                                            CIP

To
the Staff
and
the Kids
of the
Orthogenic School

This is a book about creating an environment where children will want and be able to learn. The chapters in it focus on different aspects of such a world, exploring the conditions necessary to produce a learning environment. The point of view is psychic/emotional, and therefore is not a substitute for cognitive and instructional points of view, but an addition to them.

CONTENTS

The Sonia Shankman Orthogenic School of the University of Chicago is described and explained: what it looks like, who inhabits it, and the theory that drives it. At the School all aspects, to the smallest detail, are decided upon with primary consideration for their influence on the healthful growth of its students.

Topics: diversity of influences on learning * "disturbed" as variation on normal theme * description of residents of the Orthogenic School * physical environment and its rationale * human environment (the staff) * the theory * the therapy *

The translation of psychoanalytic theory into the art of encouraging growth is exemplified. This is the theoretical perspective that underlies the Orthogenic School. The emphasis in its utilization is on what it teaches about learning and growth, more than on what it teaches about unlearning and uncovering.

Topics: misconceptions of an analytic attitude * hazards of free expression * careful listening and observation * conviction of the meaningfulness of all behavior * acceptance in the face of unacceptable behavior * hazards of encouraging transference * value of self-knowledge for the staff * value of self-acceptance for the staff *

CONTENTS

What we have learned and haven't learned about the unpleasant sine qua non of most learning is debated. No one can learn much without discipline; the question is how to develop it while developing a self-determining person.
Topics: need for discipline, internal and external measures * a clear, orderly and manageable environment * consistency of expectation * models for identification * reduced conditions of stress * understanding * ability to exercise self-control versus desire to do so * what to do while the misdeed is in process * punishment * effect on nonparticipants * matching the reaction to the psyche * pros and cons of hitting and other humane aversive techniques *

The principles and practices governing the organization and design of the classrooms of the Orthogenic School are explicated. The emphasis is on the emotional factors that are important in learning. In every aspect of classroom planning, in any setting, there is a psychological/emotional component that, if considered, enhances learning.
Topics: physical structure * temporal structure * emotional/psychic preconditions for learning * a psychic curriculum * learning to trust the teacher * being in charge of learning * safe aggressiveness * the industrious self * subject matter that has psychic appeal *

Some typical psychological problems confronting teachers in their efforts to teach in a variety of settings are discussed. Issues relate to other typical adult/child relationships. Emphasis is on dealing with emotional aspects of interaction and on emotional factors to be considered in curriculum selection.
Topics: characteristics of Orthogenic School teacher * interference with understanding * on being insulted * reexamining routine assumptions * standing in the child's shoes * clarifying goals * selecting psychologically appropriate learning experiences *

CONTENTS

ACKNOWLEDGEMENTS

Since I write with examples, I would like to express my deep appreciation for those who provide them, particularly the staff and students of the Orthogenic School. Perhaps more profoundly, I want to express my appreciation for the intense support provided by that staff and those students in their intense, interdependent, and open involvement. During those years when we were much too personally involved, worked much too long, much too hard, and for much too little pay, there were a number of people who were talented beyond their titles and enabled me to run the School because of the depth of their commitment and their assumption of very major responsibilities not formally allocated. Margie Allen, Mary Margaret Bell, Leslie Cleaver, Sandy Donaldson, Marilyn Garner, Katherine Hart, Carol Israel, Linda Kostamo, Kathy Lubin, Julie Newman, and Mary Schwartz were especially sustaining both to me and to the School.

The bricks and mortar, and the idea of an Orthogenic School to help "problem" kids, have been in place since about 1915, put there mainly through the efforts of Dr. Josephine Young and the financial support of Elizabeth McCormick. The Orthogenic School was originally part of Rush Medical School; since about 1930, it has been part of the University of Chicago. Bruno Bettelheim became its principal in 1944, so that by 1952 the "school" that I came to, lived with, grew with, and to some degree changed, was his. The extent to which his ideas pervade my account of the School can perhaps be imagined when one knows that we worked very closely together for fourteen years. In subsequent years I made changes both inadvertently and deliberately, but the brilliant basis of the enterprise was his.

I also want to thank the many people of the University of

ACKNOWLEDGEMENTS

Chicago who treated the Orthogenic School and its inhabitants in a very special way: the security police who would drive me home in the middle of the night and would help us find a missing child; the plant department which would respond cheerfully to our calls for emergency repairs; the engineer who, when his fellow workers were on strike against the university, convinced them not to picket the School; Margaret Fallers, who was always there when I needed her; and the list could go on, it seems, almost to infinity.

There were many people not physically at the School who were enabling of our work. The families of our children, who had the faith to put those dearest to them in our hands, provided the essential support for our work in their cooperation with our approach. The women of the Foundation for Emotionally Disturbed Children, with their wonderful thrift shop, provided significant financial support, friendship, and a certain kind of sustaining admiration for what we were doing. My sisters and brothers-in-law, brother and sister-in-law provided me with the security of their love for and pride in me. And I am grateful to my son because, throughout those years when I worked longer hours than any of the other mothers, he always acted as though he thought I was a good mother, doing work of which he was proud.

I could not have written this book without Dr. Frank Lani. After sharing responsibility with me for two years as Associate Director, he took over the running of the School so that I could take a sabbatical year, during which I did most of the writing. I could do so in peace, without worrying about the children, because I knew that he was. I continue to be grateful to him as he continues to run the School, under my critical eye, while I have the pleasure of watching it both stay the same and grow.

INTRODUCTION

I have spent by now many years of my life encouraging minds to grow that have been frightened and inhibited, and many years teaching others to do the same. The main location for this endeavor has been the Sonia Shankman Orthogenic School of the University of Chicago, where I was a counselor and assistant to Bruno Bettelheim for thirteen years and then myself Director for another fifteen. During this period the School was the cloistered world for thirty to fifty-five young people at a time, who had come or been brought there because of their inability to successfully navigate in the normal world, in hopes that we would be able to help them to learn to do so. They were called severely emotionally disturbed in general, and in particular such things as psychotic, schizophrenic, borderline, autistic, severely neurotic, behavior-disordered, developmentally disordered, anorexic, minimally brain damaged, and impossible. We created a world for them based on our understanding of the theory of psychoanalytic ego psychology, on anything else that any of us might know, and on the dictates of our hearts.

As I pause to reflect on these years, I am both confident and skeptical of what I think I know. Assessing and measuring success in this kind of intense human endeavor is at best a flawed science, yet we have reason to believe that what we have done has had meritorious enough consequences to warrant both its exploration and its dissemination. In the ten-year period from 1972 to 1982, of the sixty young people who left the School, nine have completed some college work and twenty-five others have been graduated from college. Of these, fourteen went on to complete postgraduate degrees and four were elected to Phi Beta Kappa. These statistics by no means indicate that our methods were successful with all of our students, nor that our treatment is the treatment of choice for all severly disturbed youngsters; but it does indicate that whatever we did in regard to the nurturing of their minds is worth exploring, since all of these young people were total failures in the world when they came to our door.

This book has a twofold purpose: to present our approach and its rationale in regard to the education of our young people, and to present my ideas regarding the application of principles evolved from our work to other areas of education. My hope, of course, is that this presentation might be of some use to others who strive for similar goals.

Since my view of emotional disturbance has always been that it is a variation on a normal theme, it has been my conviction that what we learn in intensive work with disturbed youngsters has much wider applicability. I have had opportunity to test this hypothesis in a variety of situations. These include several years of work with preschoolers and their teachers, work with teachers of students of various ages and capabilities, and the raising of my own child. The lessons learned have been extremely useful to me and others.

Because youngsters at the School are both extremely sensitive and extremely fragile, it is critical that we pay attention to all details of their life. Our focus is on understanding those factors that relate to growth and learning: what facilitates and what interferes. What we thereby learn to do to facilitate such growth and learning in fragile youngsters can be usefully applied to other settings: in classrooms for other fragile and even not-so-fragile youngsters; in various living groups such as boarding schools and camps; in play and other recreational groups for normal youngsters; and even in families.

The Orthogenic School and its work have been described in detail by Bettelheim at earlier periods in its history: in 1950 in *Love Is Not Enough,*[1] in 1955 in *Truants from Life,*[2] in 1967 in *The Empty Fortress,*[3] and in 1974 in *A Home for the Heart.*[4] As might be expected, the School has both changed and remained the same since then. Any entity that does not evolve becomes stagnant. Bettelheim has had a great influence on my thinking. I owe him particular thanks for introducing me to the world of the unconscious, knowledge of which has facilitated in me a deepened respect for the minds of others and a more thorough mastery of my own. Though I have come to differ with him on some issues, I continue to admire his ability to have created an environment that pervasively reflects concern and respect for even the most aberrant and bizarre individuals.

The focus in the chapters that follow will be on the educational aspect of the School, which has not heretofore been fully presented. However, to make understandable the context in which the education takes place, I will be describing the School, the kind of people who inhabit it, and some of its basic philosophy. I will also present my conception of psychoanalytic ego psychology, which has been most influenced by some of the work of David Rapaport.[5] The presentation is not for the purpose of advancing theory, nor of presenting the *true* theory, but of explicating the rationale behind our organization of life at the School and action in it. It has now been fifteen years since the publication of a book on the Orthogenic School. The description undertaken herein will, therefore, also serve to address the changes that have taken place. Those changes have been the result of a mix of factors: developments in the field, reexamination of our own practices, reflections of personality, and the influence of changing mores.

ONE

A Place to Grow

When any of us try to remember how we have learned, when we have learned, why we have learned, we have to recognize a multitude of diverse factors. When I was a child, I loved the comfortable little library where I went from one end of the shelf of beginning readers to the other; but when I was a college instructor, the comfort of a balmy spring evening, to which we had escaped from a claustrophobic classroom, was enough to divert my whole class from the psychology I was trying to teach. In high school I spent my after-school hours studying Hebrew and the Bible to honor my Jewish heritage and compete with my older brother in a world that did not yet recognize feminine rights. But in college I could not put my mind to physics in a class of five hundred young men and five young women. When I was growing up math had an intrinsic fascination for me, no matter who taught it. But the love of Latin had to be kindled by the lectures of a poetic Professor Finley at Harvard.

Such diversity seems to be not unique to me, but quite common, and leads to a notion that has been substantiated in all that I've read and witnessed throughout my life: that all aspects of life impinge on and influence what one learns. The ideal educational enterprise would, therefore, be one in which all aspects of the milieu in which the learner exists are thoughtfully examined. This is, of course, not a new notion; one might recognize its elements in Plato. I do not propose to have attained the ideal, but I do propose to discuss those aspects on which we have for many years concentrated and which we believe to have contributed substantially to the development in our youngsters of the ability to learn. Those aspects are the structure of the physical environment and the nature of the human environment.

CHAPTER ONE

I start, then, with a description of the general milieu that we have created for those children whom we teach—teach in general to live and, in particular to learn. Though these young people are considered to be "disturbed" and act enough at variance from most of the population to be dubbed "abnormal," the rationale that we apply to our considerations of how to treat them is no different from that which we apply to the "normal." It has been my view, substantiated by clinical experience, that for the most part the difference in treatment is one of intensity rather than kind. For example, I will later endeavor to make the point that children learn to read more easily using subject matter that has psychological relevance to them. This is probably the case for all children, but most children can, nonetheless, learn to read from any kind of nonsense. Though I had gone to great lengths to find appropriate material for a nonreader, when my son complained about the silliness of his beginning reading book, I told him to stop complaining and learn to read so then he could choose what he wanted. (He did.) It is only for children who have severe difficulty that the subject matter might become a determining factor in their learning to read. Thus, the principles behind what we do are applicable generally; how critical they might be to learning and growth depends on the individuals who are learning and growing.

The Sonia Shankman Orthogenic School of the University of Chicago is a residential treatment institution for the rehabilitation of severely disturbed children and adolescents. It is referred to by those who inhabit it, both staff and students, as "the school." How this practice came into being I don't recall. It is, nonetheless, an appropriate reflection of the process that takes place there, which is primarily a learning, growing process.

The young people who come to the School, though referred by a variety of agencies, all have severe psychiatric diagnoses. They have in common an inability to manage in any of the arenas of life: in their families, in their schools, or with their peers. They also have in common the need for a constantly supportive environment in order to learn to manage. The cause of their problems is neither intellectual nor organic. They are all in sound health with no physical impairment or intellectual deficiency. We conceptualize the problem as that of "ego deficit with undetermined etiology." Though some of our students had traumatic early lives, by no means did all of them. Why life has proved to be too much for these younsters we may speculate, but we do not know. We have found that by living it with them, and teaching them how to live it themselves, we can help them to develop the strength to master its demands and enjoy its pleasures.

We have occasionally had a student with a specific biochemical deficit that has been managed by medication. In general, however, we take students for whom there is no known medical treatment. We do not use psychotropic medication as part of our treatment (though we have used it from time to time when indicated for temporary conditions) and, therefore, do not accept students for whom that is a treatment of choice. There is, of course, a large number of students for whom there is a difference of opinion as to whether pharmacological treatment is the treatment of choice. We leave this decision to the referring physician or team.

Though in the introduction I presented the array of diagnoses that our young people come with, I never like to describe them according to diagnosis. The reasons for this dislike are, first, that diagnoses tend to vary with the diagnoser or the diagnostic group, and, second, that a diagnosis cannot take into account all aspects of a person. All our students have diagnoses from the referring agencies. Often the diagnosis tends to present a picture of more disturbance than actually exists. The issue is that in giving diagnoses the referring person is emphasizing the sickness, while in our therapeutic endeavors, from the start we emphasize the health. We focus our attention and energy on it so that we can do whatever we can to help it grow. I often remember Bettelheim's admonition to a graduate when he presented him with our parting gift, a light meter: "Remember, always measure the light and not the shadows."

When a child or adolescent is referred to us, the parents and referring agency see no less drastic an alternative than residiential treatment, with very little contact with family or friends. At that point, the youngster is usually manifesting most disturbed symptoms. If we are successful in our initial contacts, the youngster is able to reveal to us underlying strengths, which form the basis of what I call a "therapeutic alliance." Teenagers are often in rebellion against their parents and unable to form a therapeutic attachment on an outpatient basis. One teenager had let it be known to those around her that she had had hallucinatory experiences, but she would not talk with anyone about them. Since she had not let anyone know that she knew exactly when they had started, was aware of their unreality, had some understanding of their cause, wanted to understand more, and was terrified by them, the symptom was interpreted in the most serious way by the referring psychiatrist. However, she was able in our first interviews to talk more fully about such events, probably because in coming to us she was able to recognize her plight, and she had some hope that we offered an opportunity for some solution. She thus exhibited a more healthy aspect of herself (a manifestation of an "observing ego") and we, therefore, formed a more optimistic view. Similarly, a very disruptive, aggressive youngster had been afraid to confide in anyone how bad he felt about his aggressiveness and how desperate he was to control it. Since he saw relief in the prospect of coming to the School, he was able to reveal these sentiments to us in early interviews. Without the benefit of the child's point of view, the child seems only to be unmanageable, and a more severe diagnosis is given.

In our procedures, we try to focus on the elements of strength in the child's psyche and tend to accept for admission those who, despite severe diagnoses, have clear strengths. A reflection of this approach is that in the first visits of parent and child together, I have always talked with the child first. In these discussions I have always asked for the child's view of the problem and have been very direct about the reasons for considering placement.

Two major elements in our decision as to whether to accept a child are, first, whether we believe that we can establish a therapeutic alliance and, second, whether the child has a desire to get better. We are probably not as demanding in our criteria regarding the ability to establish a therapeutic alliance as many professionals in less encompassing settings, since we are able to be more continually attentive to our clients. That is, when the child is living with us, if the desire to get better manifests itself at 5:00 in the afternoon or 8:00 in the morning, there is someone around who can respond and encourage it. Furthermore, it can manifest itself in many ways other than the direct "talking about one's problems," such as asking for comfort, responding to a staff member's efforts to teach self-control, or being empathic with a needy dorm mate. We have more opportunity to develop a therapeutic alliance and to respond to even a very slight desire to get better than do those who practice a more time-and-place-limited type of therapy. With this expectation, we can base our initial judgement on even very small signs of ability to ally and desire to get better. Younger children cannot always express this desire verbally so we note other indications of their responsiveness in action, such as their attentiveness to us and their ability to accept needed help. Older students can in our first meeting let us know explicitly that they want to change. These two criteria lead to a selection of young people with some degree of positive attitude and therapeutic mores.

Children are referred to the Orthogenic School from all over. The children referred are in quite desperate straits. Their desperation arises in part from the distress of their disturbance and in part from the inability of their environment to provide the intensity and variety of supports necessary for the alleviation of that distress. A family situation, for example, can be such that it is unmanageable, with any amount of family therapy. A family with only one child can often provide more tolerance and support for the child's difficult behavior than a family with other younger, vulnerable children. Or there may not be available in the community the necessary all-encompassing, intensive services needed. Referrals and our screening procedures have led over the years to a population of youngsters with a wide variety of characteristics. They have ranged in age from five to twenty-five and in demeanor from those with bizarre mannerisms to those who look indistinguishable from their age mates in any ordinary setting. In their conversational ability our youngsters have similarly ranged from those who have little speech and unusual speech patterning, to those who are bright and engaging in their social contacts. They have had some exceptional talents, in art, in physical agility, and in mathematics, for example.

At any given moment, to someone walking around the School, our youngsters would seem to be "an ordinary bunch of kids." On staying around for a while, that person would see a range of behavior that would be unexpected and remarkable in "an ordinary bunch of kids" going from bizarre and primitive through ordinary to most sensitive and sophisticated. One teacher in the course of a day will hold a girl to prevent her from hurting herself, encourage a boy to refrain from making a nasty remark, and conduct a class discussion on a recent play being performed by the university's Court Theatre.

In our efforts to help these young people, we practice our view of psychoanalytically oriented milieu therapy. This means that ideally all aspects of the environment are designed to be therapeutic and that the design of the environment is based on psychoanalytic concepts, with particular reference to ego issues. The use of "ego" is not in the most common dictionary-definition sense, but is my version of the psychoanalytic sense. I mean simply that part of the psyche that "keeps the show on the road." It is that part of the psyche that usually feels like "I", that part that manages our inner turmoil and enables us to satisfy our desires and meet the demands that are made on us by the external world. An ego that is weak is not able to manage inner turmoil, to satisfy needs, or to conform to external demands. In order for it to develop that ability it needs exercise in small doses and, therefore, a modified environment. In fulfilling its tasks the normal, healthy ego develops various mechanisms and has at its disposal various functions, such as intelligence, perception, and motility. The better these are developed, the stronger the ego. The young people who come to us all suffer from ego deficits; they are able to integrate neither experiences nor the various aspects of their personalities. They need almost constant ego support and, ideally, a total environment, physical and human, that is designed to accommodate them, both so that they can master it and so that it can provide the appropriate challenges for growth.[1]

Psychoanalytically oriented milieu therapy at the Orthogenic School consists of a physical environment, a human environment, a theory, and a therapy. The physical environment is a school that we try to make as warm, beautiful, safe, and manageable as possible. The human environment is the staff. The theory that informs our action in, and arrangement of, these environments is that of psychoanalytic ego psychology, modernized with some more recent psychoanalytic concepts. The therapy is the gradual and consistent education of the ego. This involves the modification of, on the one hand, the external environment and, on the other, the internal environment, to suit the capacity of the weak or malformed ego. It involves at the same time the provision of ego support to help the student develop the various ego functions.

In constructing and arranging the physical environment, we try to consider the messages we want to convey and the messages that various selections and arrangements do convey. The three aspects that we believe to be of greatest importance for a school like ours to emphasize are: that it is safe; that it is for its inhabitants; and that those inhabitants are very worthy persons. Since our students typically come to us beset by overwhelming anxiety, feeling always at risk of some degree of destruction either at the hands of themselves or others, safety is a major issue. These young people, though most often not physically abused, usually feel untrusting of the intentions of others. Further, their experience has been that their own efforts frequently bring bad consequences to themselves. For many, these anxieties about emotional harm are often translated into anxiety about physical harm. To make an environment safe for children who are sometimes destructive to themselves and others often requires some ingenuity. We tend to provide safety by human supervision rather than by physical isolation and have constructed an environment that makes this easily possible. The arrangement of space, for example, tends to be of such a dimension that a group of seven or so can have comfortable movement, but be always visible to a responsible person. Privacy is, of course, an important issue. However, the child who is afraid that a hand might reach up from a toilet bowl, or the teenager who is intermittently beset by impulses to scratch herself, is more in need of compassionate protective company than lonely and potentially frightening privacy.

At the same time, the safety has to be provided in a way that does not imply that those in safekeeping are bad. Furnishings must be attractive and useful as well as sturdy. The appropriate selection of furnishings requires the time and thoughtful care of the people who know and understand best the needs of our youngsters. Since our students typically have felt that they have lived in a world that is not for them, in a world in which they have failed, it also has to be apparent that the School is designed for its inhabitants, and that those inhabitants are considered to be very valuable. The School is, therefore, a very attractive place, with works of art, good furnishings, and colorful appointments.

A youngster coming to the Orthogenic School lives in one of six very large, bright dormitories, with five or six other young people. Each dormitory is furnished differently. We try to make it comfortable, attractive, and, most importantly, to make it feel like it belongs to each youngster as a home. In each dormitory there is a locked closet where anything that is necessary for use but potentially dangerous (e.g., scissors, nail polish) is locked up. The children have many personal items in their areas, so that the rooms have the feeling of ordinary, cluttered, young peoples' rooms. They are free to arrange their areas however they wish, with posters, paintings, stuffed animals, mementoes, weather-predicting paraphernalia, as long as there is nothing that is dangerous or frightening. In addition, the students make as many decisions as possible about their living environment. When the rooms are painted, they choose the colors. When we got new silverware, they voted on the pattern. When we had a sculpture made for an outdoor fountain, they talked with the sculptor about their ideas.

This dormitory is their base of operations. Each child's area has a bed, dresser, toy chest, and rug. It is inviolate; no one can touch it without permission, though it is rare that a child would not give permission to have the bed made. It is extremely important to them that this injunction be respected. For children who need much external control in order to manage their lives, it is especially important that any area where they can safely exercise their independent control be given the utmost respect and encouragement to develop. Furthermore, many view their bed and belongings as extensions of themselves, so that any intrusion into their areas or thoughtless handling of their belongings can be experienced as an insufferable violation of a delicate boundary.

There is also a group area, with a round table and chairs. There are group belongings and shelves for them: games, art material, food-making equipment, and other paraphernalia necessary for shared interests. The group congregates around the table for snacks, conversation, and group projects. There is, therefore, an individual haven and a group haven. This arrangement permits a child to be somewhat isolated yet still part of whatever transpires in the group. It also permits the supervising person (the counselor) to have some awareness of the tone and state of each of the group members at all times without necessarily having a direct or obvious interaction. A brilliant but isolated young man, a graduate of the School, when interviewed during his graduate college years told me that one of the most important aspects of the School was this provision of the presence of others. Though he spent much of his time with a book on his bed, the continual presence of the other boys and the staff enabled him to be a part of a personal atmosphere for which he could not himself reach out.

The personal and group possessions are to some extent selected by the children and to some extent selected by the staff. The selections by the staff are most often purposeful, to convey some notion of the directions of growth that they wish to encourage. A stiff, schizophrenic girl was given a print of Renoir's bather when she began to have some greater ability to enjoy her body. She hung it on her wall where it served as a constant encouragement. There are many books at the School and a great variety of equipment, reflecting our efforts to broaden the vistas of the students and to entice them into constructive activity.

The next most utilized room is, of course, the dining room, which is designed to make meal times as comfortable and sociable as possible. Students eat breakfast and dinner with their dormitory group and counselor at their table. They eat lunch with their classroom group and teacher at their table in the same dining room. Meals are served family style. There is a staff table in the dining room where the staff who live at the School or are for any reason at the School at a meal time have their meals. We use china, glassware, and attractive serving pieces. We believe, with Montessori, that if one gives children things of beauty that need care, they will feel that beauty is for them and will learn to be careful.[2] The whole school coming together several times a day contributes to the feeling of unity that is very important at the School. This unity provides an emotional support and an avenue for the development of common mores. The Director's or Associate Director's presence and interaction with staff and students serves as a demonstration of some of these mores. When the Director steps in or refrains from stepping in, everyone can see what "goes" and what "doesn't go." Everyone can see that respectful behavior is expected from everyone, and that personal pain is understood.

The School occupies about one-quarter of a city block: half of this is taken up by the building, and the remainder is outdoor play area. A child can stay on the grounds of the School and yet experience a wide variety of environmental textures. There are approximately ten common rooms, each one distinct from the other and each one with distinct character provided by some built-in feature. Since the young people that we deal with tend to be in a chaotic state internally, they are able to function better when the environment is structured for them. Most of the rooms, therefore, are very clearly defined by the way they look. The living room has soft chairs, gold wallpaper, ceramic chandeliers, a record player, a television, and bookshelves with games and books. The recreation room has a concrete floor, a pool table, and a ping pong table. The outdoor areas are divided by hedges and are also clearly defined, with grassy hills for quiet talks and a flat field for baseball or jogging. There is little question as to what is appropriate to do in each space.

Session rooms are furnished as rather typical play therapy rooms; each is designed to be a private space where a child can meet regularly with a staff member. The counselors have private living rooms both in areas adjacent to and at a distance from the dormitory areas. These locations reflect both the desirability of closeness to the children at times when staff members are not officially working and the importance of being able to have sufficient distance from the work and the children during a substantial part of that time. The offices are spaces that have been converted from rooms in the oldest part of the building.

I began this description of the physical environment with generalizations about that part of it in which the children spend the most time. I will end with a description of the first physical impressions of the School. One enters what was once a minister's home, through a yellow door, past a blue Spanish door laden with painted fruit and angels. One then turns left to the living room and sits on a very soft sofa or chair and looks around at an old-fashioned, somewhat dilapidated doll house, a wooden seahorse from a merry-go-round on Cape Cod, an elaborate bishop's chair from one of the storehouses of the university, a cradle from Germany containing a somewhat homely rag doll, and a curious table and chair with dragon heads on them. If one is either a parent or a child coming to the School for the first time, the environment of these first moments has silently conveyed a message.

How might we describe the message? All of the funishings were chosen with love and care, chosen because someone thought they would be fun or pretty or good for children at the School to have. A parent gave us the doll house and a student painted it; the head of buildings and grounds at the university found the bishop's chair and thought we would like it; Bettelheim bought the seahorse and the cradle on his travels; and some wealthy benefactor donated the table and chair. All of these people wanted to do something for children who were suffering, and thought they would enjoy and appreciate these lovely antiques. So, the message is one of care, respect, and concern. This seems a most appropriate message for a family to receive when its child is about to enter residential treatment.

The members of the human environment who have the potential for the strongest therapeutic effect are those who are with the children the most, the counselors and the teachers. Each dormitory group has three counselors. They divide the week, except for class time and sleeping time, among themselves, so that at any given time one of the three is with the group. They are responsible for all aspects of the children's lives, so they spend individual time with children going shopping, going to the dentist, the doctor, or wherever else is necessary, and doing things just for fun. Counselors are usually recent college graduates who come to the School because they are interested in working with needy youngsters and in having the kind of learning experience offered. They tend to be idealistic people. Most are committed to the helping professions, but others simply want to do something helpful for a while and to learn about people. In the forties and fifties the counselors were predominantly young women, choosing to spend some time before starting their own families in helping others and hoping to learn things that would be useful to them later in raising their children. By the seventies and eighties there had been a change in the typical motivation of applicants, in keeping with the change in society. More men began applying for the positions, and the women tended to have more professional goals; frequently they planned to become clinical psychologists. During these years we have developed a program for counselors that has a more formal academic component. Though there tends to be a consistency of age and educational level, there is a diversity of geographical background and educational training. People come from all over the country and from a variety of liberal arts colleges and programs. There have also usually been at any given time a couple of people from abroad, who have come because of the reputation of the School. The atmosphere among the counselors is of intense involvement and intense commitment to the students and to their own learning and growth. It is not uncommon that counselors consider their experience at the School as among the most difficult, yet most rewarding and enriching, of their lives.

Children are all in class from 9:00 A.M. to 3:00 P.M., five days a week, with five or six classmates and their teacher, who teaches them all subjects, for several years in a row. The teachers have at least bachelor's degrees and, most commonly, special education certification. A number of times over the years there have been teachers with doctorates interested in the opportunity to work directly with severely disturbed youngsters. Teachers have ranged in age from their early twenties to retirement age, and in previous teaching experience from only a year or two to many years. They are all strongly committed to teaching, but enjoy the work at the

School because of the possibility it affords to gain and use knowledge of the whole child and to be engaged in a multidimensional way with their students. They also enjoy being able to be responsible for the construction of the class—its curriculum and activities—with the advice and support of their colleagues. The teachers work longer and more contiguous teaching hours than most teachers, and they regularly attend after-class meetings. They consider their long hours a worthwhile exchange for the ability to have a stronger impact on the growth of their children.

The counselors and teachers comprise the core of the therapeutic milieu. The ultimate authority and responsibility for the nature of this milieu lies in the hands of the Director with, in the later years of the period described, the Associate Director. They are psychologists with many years of experience with disturbed young people in residential settings. It is their task both to guide the treatment and to manage the milieu. This entails an active participation in the life of the School, including being present at important though inconvenient times. Some of the most significant experiences for some students have transpired between them and the Director during sleepless or otherwise disturbed nights. And the quality of a holiday celebration, for children so prone to feel deserted and unworthy, is much enhanced by the presence of the head of the enterprise.

The task of the Director also entails intervention, both to exercise authority in the control of behavior and to exercise skill in resolving problems, through understanding and sensitivity at critical times. A teenager, somewhat prone to delinquency, once said to me, "I will do what you or Dr. B. [it was the first year of my tenure and Bettelheim was still officially the Director] tell me even when I don't agree because I think you have my best interest at heart. But I won't listen to Q [one of his counselors] because he doesn't." I believe that authority exercised in the judicious combination of understanding and sensitivity leads to the kind of respect and support for authority expressed in the first part of the young man's statement. That is, he could follow the law even when he neither understood nor agreed with it because, out of his experience, he believed that it was ultimately motivated by a

concern for his best interest. (It was also our task to understand why he did not trust his counselor. If his mistrust had
validity, we would attempt to educate the counselor; if it did
not, then we would attempt to help the boy with his misper-
ception.)

The Director's task also entails active participation in the
teaching and support of the staff, both in their learning a
therapeutic mode and in their developing the ability to manage the emotions that working with difficult and demanding
people invariably evokes.

The directors are assisted in their task of therapeutic direction by two consultant psychoanalysts, who each come to the
School once a week. At this time the consultant meets individually with one of the students and then meets with the staff
about the child. For this meeting each person who works directly with the child prepares a report. One of the consultants
is a child analyst in private practice, and one is an analyst
responsible for the psychiatric unit of a large hospital. Some of
the students feel that the analysts are of direct help to them,
but actually their main purpose is consultation for the staff and
Directors. By having analysts as our consultants, we insure
input of an analytic approach. Though none of our students
are in analysis, we make use of analytic insights and theory to
better understand them and to know how to structure their
experiences and environment.

The Directors were for many years assisted in their task of
teaching and support to the staff by senior counselors. As
counselors gained in experience, they would share their experience with younger staff in countless hours of discussion.
They would also make themselves available to their newer
coworkers for crisis intervention. These senior counselors
worked long and hard with no reward other than the personal
gratification they gained. In more recent years the task of guid-
ing the counselors has been undertaken by three mental health
professionals, who are either social workers or psychologists
with many years of experience in milieu therapy. This kind of
experience enables them to provide truly empathic guidance.
In the management of the milieu the Directors are also assisted
by a head counselor who has had many years of experience as

a counselor. There is a good deal of flexibility in these roles, both in the mode of exercising the responsibilities resting therein, and in the possibility of reallocating those responsibilities. The organic nature of the whole requires that the personality of the person holding a position substantially influences the character and determination of the role. Furthermore, the sensitive nature of the students demands more the kind of authority that is earned by virtue of a person's interactional qualities, than the kind of authority that is assigned by role designation.

The counselors and teachers are assisted in their efforts to create an environment for growth by a variety of other workers, sometimes students from local educational institutions or training programs, and sometimes specialty teachers. The physical education teacher is always a very important part of our program, because of the importance of physical mastery and feelings of body competence to anxious youngsters. We also try to have some classes for relatively homogeneous groups of students, with subject matter selected for its benefit to them and directed toward curriculum development. Teaching this kind of class requires unusual talent; our children are difficult to manage in groups unless the leader of the group knows them very well.

At a time that seems appropriate in terms of the child's development, each child is offered individual sessions with a counselor, a teacher, or one of the mental health professionals. The purpose of these sessions varies with the individual. They are considered to be an adjunct to the core therapeutic thrust of the milieu. Sometimes the sessions provide an opportunity to concentrate on a particular kind of learning, at other times they serve to help the child feel special, and at yet other times they are utilized for quiet reflection in the presence of another. Since the early transferences that are evoked in sessions when transference is encouraged are likely to arouse feelings that are more disruptive than can be tolerated by the fragile egos of our students, we do not encourage transference. However, since in daily life transference-like phenomena very frequently occur, it is important that the staff be taught to understand it. When a child has sessions with a counselor or teacher, the counselor or teacher is closely supervised by a staff member who is experienced and well trained in both milieu and individual psychoanalytic psychotherapy.

Since the physical environment, including its nourishing elements, is considered to be such a significant part of the therapeutic milieu, those who maintain it make a vital contribution to that milieu. The cleaning and kitchen staff are important to the School and to the children, and the School and children are important to them. Though somewhat less visible, the office staff is also known and important to the children.

A strength of the School is its unity of purpose. It is possible to develop strong mores if the staff is singleminded in the support of those mores. To achieve this unity requires much consistent effort: the staff lives together, eats together, meets together, works together, and talks together. It is an intense environment, with very strong personal commitments to learning and growing. The staff forms strong attachments to their students and to each other.

As Director of this enterprise, I have organized my thinking around my understanding of the theory of psychoanalytic ego psychology. I have based my decisions regarding the arrangement and action of the above-described environment on my understanding of human beings as derived from this theory and from some more recent developments. It is not the purpose of this book to present a comprehensive statement of theory, but the following is a brief statement of what I consider to be the most important aspects of the theory for our work.[3]

Human beings are motivated by unconscious as well as conscious thoughts, feelings, and desires. An understanding of the nature of this unconscious realm is helpful in explaining contradictory or puzzling behavior and is helpful in finding avenues to communicate with people who seem incomprehensible. The unconscious consists of a conglomerate of needs and past experiences; each person's unconscious is both unique and universal. It is, of course, not possible to know the unconscious, since that is a contradiction in terms, but it is possible to make reasonable speculations about it.

A person's present state is influenced by experiences in the past. Experience in this sense is an interactive event, including the individual (both biologic and psychic) and the environment. Certain experiences in development are considered to be universal. The stages of psychosexual development, the stages of psychosocial development, and the process of separation-individuation are basic experiences that all people are considered to go through. How these stages are mastered is important in determining the kind of person an individual becomes.

A person is considered to have a certain amount of psychic energy. The theory of stages of development postulates the location of the greatest investment of this energy at the various stages. (For example, in terms of the theory of psychosexual development, the psychic energy of an infant is postulated to be focused around the mouth; therefore, the first stage is called oral). Normal development supposes a movement of this energy to different loci as a person grows. All mental activity requires expenditure of psychic energy.

The theoretical structure of the mental apparatus is considered to consist of ego, super-ego, and id. At birth all mental energy resides in the id, that part of the psyche that is comprised of instincts and primitive desires. The ego develops in interaction with the environment: it is considered to be the human's organ of adaptation. It has the task of satisfying internal demands (of the id and super-ego) and external demands of the environment. The super-ego is that part of the psyche that is comprised of the automatic commands and demands internalized from the external world. In order to perform its functions, the ego has to have a multiplicity of mechanisms. It has to have control of such processes as motility, cognition, and intelligence, and also of psychic mechanisms as defenses to protect the organism from overwhelming anxiety.

It is part of my understanding of this theory that the development of cognitive, intellectual, perceptual, and physical abilities, and the maintenance of biological health, are intrinsic to healthy ego development. An example of this is in the area of reality testing, a fairly well-known ego function, the strength of which is often used as a measure of mental health. We can define reality testing as the ability to accurately test and assess one's perception and interpretation of the world. It is the ability to recognize and accept, for example, that one has set out to climb a mountain that is higher than the height one has the stamina to reach. While the ability to make this evaluation (reality test) requires emotional strength and maturity, it requires first the ability to see clearly and to understand what one sees. It is not possible to have good reality testing without the cognitive ability to perceive well and to interpret accurately.

In terms of the foregoing brief outline, a healthy person is a person with a strong ego, able to master the demands of both inner and outer worlds. That is to say, if one can meet one's own needs and satisfy societal, familial, and environmental demands, one is healthy. A person can be as bizarre or in as much misery as can be imagined without being considered mentally ill. Most people go into therapy because they are unable to meet some aspect of these demands that they want to meet, or suffer more psychic anguish than they wish to tolerate. Such people are usually identified as being neurotic rather than mentally ill. People who require hospitalization are usually considered mentally ill. They cannot meet either internal or external demands: their behavior oversteps the bounds of external acceptability (leading to harm to themselves or others), or they are not able to meet their own needs. Our students similarly come to us because of their inability to meet these demands, because their egos are not up to the task. We consider our primary task to be the strengthening of the ego.

We believe that the ego becomes strong in its exercise. We therefore endeavor to construct an environment the demands of which can be mastered by the very fragile egos of our students. Constructing such an environment requires a knowledge of their capabilities and stage of development on every level—physical, intellectual, psychic—so that the tasks we present to develop their mastery of the world, and to enhance their skills, will be both challenging and manageable. It also requires knowledge of their psychic makeup so that we can guide them through the stages of development that they may have failed to navigate successfully, protect them from experiences that produce overwhelming anxiety, reduce conflictual issues so they can eventually have the energy to resolve them, and stimulate growth by appeal to areas where energy is invested and available.

We see the work of the Orthogenic School to be primarily an ego-educative enterprise. Perhaps that is why we call it "the School." The appellation is, perhaps, a reflection of our efforts to create a learning place, where our young people can learn to trust, learn to try, learn to play, learn to learn, and learn to live.

TWO

A Philosophy (Psychology)
in Practice

My idea of milieu therapy is that the therapy surrounds the
patient; that it pervades all aspects of life—play time, school
time, meal time, bed time, talk time. In order to achieve such a
therapeutic milieu, all participants in it (particularly the staff)
should ideally have a therapeutic attitude. And such an attitude, in a milieu that is psychoanalytically oriented, should
be, of course, psychoanalytic. Since a "psychoanalytic attitude" does not have the same meaning for everyone, in order
to clarify the nature of our therapeutic milieu I believe it necessary to elaborate on its meaning to me.

I will begin with what I do *not* mean, particularly in regard
to some misconceptions—notions that we frequently encounter people attributing to an analytic attitude. The first thing
that we do not mean is that we always encourage our children
to "express" themselves, or that we encourage and accept all
kinds of primitive and aggressive acting out. In fact, at times
we expect our children to keep quiet and *not* express their
feelings. We consider one of our most important tasks to be
that of helping them to develop self-control. In order to have
self-control, it is necessary to differentiate feeling from action,
to separate *having* feelings from talking about or acting on
them. We, furthermore, do *not* mean that we try to read the
minds of our children and offer deep interpretations relating to
sexual strivings and to conflicts from their past. And we certainly do not mean that we have our students lie down on a
couch for an hour a day. They have much need for activity, and
we hope that when they do lie down it will be to go to sleep
and not to talk to us or anyone else. These are stereotyped
ideas of some methods that, when used appropriately, are
appropriate in some particular analytic settings, effected by

people with particular skills. They are not appropriate for our setting, nor for the students that we treat.

However, there are some stereotyped ideas of analytic attitudes that are very appropriate for our setting and for the children we treat, and that are very much a part of what we mean by an application of psychoanalytic theory. These are ideas that we try to emphasize continually in our work, and they are likely to be ideas that are appropriate in many other settings.

By a psychoanalytic attitude we *do* mean that we listen to and watch very carefully what our children say and do, that we use all of our powers of empathy to understand the meaning of what they say and do, and that we make every effort to see the world from their point of view. To me these are the essential ingredients of a psychoanalytic approach. Freud, as I understand his method, listened very carefully to the productions of his patients and worked very hard to puzzle out the possible meanings of behavior that appeared inexplicable. All of his theory derived from these observations and speculations. The theory is dependent on observations and can be considered valid only if it continues to effectively explain further careful observations. In my view the success of any analytic venture depends on this very careful attentiveness and the conviction that there is logic and meaning to the productions of the person whom we are watching and to whom we are listening.

I believe that this approach has been the basis of our success in establishing contact with autistic and psychotic children and the basis of our ability to establish trust with our less severely disturbed children. Because of our conviction that their behavior is meaningful, we do not interpret the withdrawn behavior of an autistic child as a lack of any attentiveness to the world, or the productions of a psychotic child as incomprehensible bizarreness, or the acting up of a behavior-disordered child as badness. We view all of these as having meaning and purpose, and, before making efforts to change the behavior, we listen, watch, and try to understand it. Once children or adolescents feel that they are understood, or that we are very interested in understanding, they are not only relieved, but eventually they begin to be willing to explain themselves to us more, and even perhaps gradually change.

A Philosophy (Psychology) in Practice

Our attitude is not very different from the reaction of a mother to her infant. It happens frequently that a mother will see her infant's behavior as meaningful before anyone else does. When the baby smiles she thinks that it is because of her presence; when it cries she explains that it is because of a need. The pediatrician or a benevolent friend explains the behavior very differently, attributing the smile to gas pains and the cry to the baby's being spoiled. The attentive mother who sees her infant's behavior as meaningful and responds to it in those terms is more likely to have a contented baby, and one who is more likely to develop communication skills with her.

One of our boys has reminded me more than once of a night when he was twelve years old and wildly running around the School, threatening aggression to his counselor if he interfered. When he sat down for a few minutes, he told me that he was afraid of a tornado. This was not a realistic anxiety. However, explaining that to him did not help at all to alleviate the anxiety. Because of our knowledge of his history we could understand that he might have experienced his father's drunken rages as a tornado. Perhaps trying to gain mastery by an identification with his father, he was now running around the School wreaking havoc like a tornado. At this point in our relationship and in his relationship with the School, should anyone have said that, he might have been very upset, out of loyalty to his father. Though he feared his father, he also loved him and was dependent on him. It was important to convey to the boy in some way that we took his anxiety seriously and were going to try to help him with it. I told him that I could make a sign for him with an arrow saying "Tornados go that way, no tornados allowed here." He was both old and young enough to accept this: old enough to realize that tornados neither read nor obey signs, and young enough to hope that they would do both. He has recalled it as a cherished moment—because he responded to my symbolic reaffirmation that I, as Director, would continue to keep the tornado out. My response required careful attention to his words and actions and a serious effort to understand their significance.

Those who work with autistic children know that a common characteristic is the inability to make eye contact; these children never look you in the eye. In our work, it has never taken long for us to establish this eye contact, though we have never approached the issue directly. We do not even tell these children to look at us, far from insisting that they do so. I believe that the reason for our success in this area is our approach that whatever they do is meaningful and that we try to respond to their messages in terms of our understanding of that meaningfulness. When an autistic girl shredded her food into tiny pieces before eating it, making a mess all around her, we did not criticize her for it or insist that she clean it up. We put our heads together and speculated that she may not have trusted the safety of the food. This speculation had some support from her past, since her parents had gone to great lengths to hide vitamins in her cereal and candy bars. We did our best to reassure her that we would not hide anything in her food. At the same time we provided means so that the mess she created would be manageable, both for herself and those who had to live with her, for example, by having a tray on her lap when she had a snack. Her need to shred gradually was alleviated, and with this and other similar experiences her trust in us and ability to look at us grew.

The behavior of psychotic people can often be understood through careful observation and efforts to understand. We have had with us a psychotic adolescent girl who had a major difficulty with the issue of loss because of the accidental death of a favored sister. After being with us for a short while she began to make a "film." This project entailed mostly writing lists of names and places on paper in apparently incomprehensible ways, with strange formations and designs. Her teacher figured out that these lists were somehow combinations of meaningful people and places from her past. The girl took to carrying the materials for her film around with her in shopping bags, which became more and more voluminous as the pages of the film grew. The film began to include all kinds of objects of various meaning, most often incomprehensible to anyone else. Since we believed that this film was an effort to emotionally establish her attachments to her past and to organize these attachments, we provided her with material for her production and helped her carry it around. Her enterprising teacher even found a way to project her film for the other girls in her group, when she wanted to use it as a birthday activity.

He used an overhead projector, so that the visual reproduction of an object placed on a table could be shown on an opposite wall. Gradually the number of items necessary for her to carry around decreased, until it was necessary only for her to carry colored writing and drawing markers. We suspected that these were a representation of her attachment to her teacher. This favored teacher left the School, and our speculation was supported when on the first day of her class with the new teacher, she asked him if he would get her the same kind of markers that her former teacher had supplied. Though it is very difficult definitely to confirm the effects of any particular action—life and human beings being so complex—we believe that her ability to utilize this kind of transitional object was helpful in her working through the issue of separation and loss. Her progress with this issue was such that when I told the students of the School that I would be away for a year she wanted, like the others, to have the opportunity to talk with me about it alone in my office. At that time she was able to say that she was sad that I was going because she liked me, but that she wasn't so sad because she knew that I would be back.

These have been some examples of the way in which we in our work assume an analytic attitude, by paying careful attention and giving deep respect to the words and actions of those in our care, trying to listen, watch, and understand, so that we can see the world through the eyes of our children.

We do not believe that the technique of traditional psychoanalysis is the treatment of choice for our severely emotionally disturbed children and adolescents. But there are some principles inherent in that technique that we do find applicable to our work with these youngsters, most notably, a safe environment and an atmosphere of attentiveness and acceptance. Traditional psychoanalysis takes place within a very clearly defined setting, within a clearly, even rigidly, defined time frame, and with clearly established rules and expectations. Within such a setting, as an analysand one is free to be oneself, with the knowledge that there will be no bad effects from whatever one might say or think. The limits set guarantee that there will be no destructive action, since there is virtually no action at all. In application to the situation of our children and adolescents, who we want to be able to be themselves, this principle means that it is necessary for them to have a very safe, clearly structured environment, with definite limits and definite rules and expectations. When it is desirable to encourage self-expression (as it very often is), it is important to make clear that self-expression is limited to ways that will not be hurtful to people.

Within this very safe setting, attentiveness and acceptance are to me critical elements. The most traditional analyst is expected to be listening and noncritical. With our young people these attitudes are also essential. One young man once told me that he could not stand it when I was critical of him. Until he came to the School he had always believed that he was a rotten kid. His experience at the School had begun to convince him that this was not true, that he did some rotten things but that he himself, perhaps, was not rotten. But when I criticized him it made him feel that I believed it, too, and so maybe he really was just a rotten kid. Since this was a boy who frequently engaged in very disruptive, aggressive, self-centered behavior, I was very much surprised and moved by this confession of sensitivity and, as I recall, made only a somewhat tongue-tied expression of sympathy. The purpose of his statement was probably twofold. On the one hand he probably wanted to convince me not to criticize him; and on the other, he probably wanted to explain why he had had a violently negative reaction to my criticism. It was a very clear statement of the importance of our conveying again and again, through words and repeated kindness, no matter what our youngsters do, that we care for and respect them and view those destructive actions (which we impede, outlaw, and criticize) as their misguided attempts to improve their lot in life. That he had to some extent received the message was evidenced in his statement, that he continued to receive the message was evidenced in his continued gradual progress. Having come to the School unable to function in any school setting and unable to be tolerated in his family, when he left us he entered a competitive college in another part of the country.

Maintaining such an attitude of acceptance is much easier said than done, as is creating a safe environment for disorganized children and rebellious adolescents. Some aspects of our approach have already been discussed. We, for example,

A PHILOSOPHY (PSYCHOLOGY) IN PRACTICE

try to arrange for destructive children by having nothing around them that is irreplaceable or easily destroyed. We can then afford to maintain the stance that human beings are more important than material goods. In this way we can emotionally be truly accepting and understanding of a child's destructiveness. As a child grows stronger, we change the expectations and have more serious consequences for infractions of rules. In the course of his residence at the School, the young man to whom I referred destroyed furniture, locks, doors, and other goods, which we replaced. In such instances it can be a very serious problem for the staff to be able to be very clearly critical of a child's actions and very clearly accepting of the child. I believe that the most difficult part is not so much that children do things for which they need to be criticized, but that because they do them so frequently and with such intensity, we may begin to believe that they really are rotten kids. This difficulty is perhaps one of the most compelling reasons for there to be very strong staff mores of understanding and a continuing pursuit of that understanding, so that we are mutually supported in maintaining a view of even the worst-acting youngster as a person of value.

For people who are with such children for long stretches of time (our counselors and teachers), to maintain an attitude of acceptance requires a great deal of help and support. For example, when a fifteen-year-old came up from class one day and asked for his allowance, his counselor told him that he would have to wait ten minutes until she had time to go to her room and get it. The boy had a tantrum, calling his counselor names and accusing her of being totally against him. Since the counselor felt that she was complying with his request and doing something to please him, it was not possible for her to understand or accept his outrage and verbal abuse. She complained to the Director (who was making rounds) about the disrespectful and inappropriate behavior of the boy, concluding that he should not be allowed to go out because of it. The Director reviewed the situation with the counselor, and they reconstructed the boy's point of view. He had asked earlier for his allowance. He had been waiting for a while to buy the item he was going out for, and was afraid he would miss a friend if he delayed his excursion. The counselor had been very busy

28

and so had forgotten to bring the allowance into the dormitory earlier. To the egocentric youngster this forgetfulness could only be construed as interference with his heart's desire. In the intensity of the moment the counselor was not able to sort this out; with the support of another staff member, she could. As soon as she approached the boy with an apology for forgetting his allowance, and sympathy for the incurred delay, he dropped his aggressive demeanor and was apologetic for his disrespectful treatment of her. Her acceptance was not of his abusive behavior but of his hurt feelings. When he felt this, he could join her in her criticism of the abusive behavior.

I would like to note that, while it may be true that the intensity of attentiveness and staff availability that I describe are luxuries that not everyone can afford, the degree of reactivity of our young people is of an intensity that is very unusual. Therefore, if our attitudes are effective with them when intensely applied, they can be effective with others at a less intense level. I believe that the principles of attitude are not luxuries, but effective tools in any situation.

While the safe, consistent, attentive, and accepting environment is of utmost importance, there are other elements in the classic analytic situation that are very different from what we practice with our students. The analysand is instructed to free-associate. Thus primary or primitive processes are encouraged, which often lead to a reawakening of memories and feelings from the past, feelings that are often disorganized and painful. To be able to tolerate this experience and eventually make use of it to understand oneself and to reorganize and reintegrate at a higher level requires not only the safe structure of the analytic situation, but also a strong and well-developed personality structure. Since our young people do not have the necessary strength of personality structure, if these primitive processes are encouraged it is most likely to be debilitating, like raging waters beating against a weak dam. Thus the naive staff member's well-meaning encouragement to self-expression can often be devastating.

Another important difference is in the use of transference-like phenomena. I define that term very broadly and loosely as referring to the reexperiencing in the present of elements of relationships from the past, so that the person attributes to

29

someone in the present aspects of significant figures of the past. In the analytic situation transference to the analyst is examined, understood, and resolved; the analysand is then free to find new ways of relating. In our situation, we make use of the positive aspects of transference-like phenomena to influence our young people in their attitude and approach to life. We also use the development of positive relationships as demonstration that negative transference-like expectations of relationships are not valid. When a prepubertal boy developed a positive transference-like relationship to his male teacher, based on his idealized relationship with his father, the teacher used this relationship to encourage his learning, strengthen his desire to control his acting out, and adopt a somewhat more reasonable view of his female counselor, to whom he had developed a negative transference-like relationship.

I have by no means, of course, covered all aspects of analytic treatment. What I have tried to discuss are some of the salient issues that I find most often misunderstood in efforts to more broadly apply psychoanalytic theory.

The foregoing discussion has been about attitudes toward those we treat. An area that I believe to be of greatest importance and inestimable value to the worker in a psychoanalytic approach is self-knowledge. Anyone who has worked with severely disturbed individuals is familiar with the onslaught of emotion—primitive, complex, ambivalent—which such individuals present. It is our belief that successfully dealing with this onslaught can contribute significantly to the professional development of the worker and to the patient's course of treatment. Whether the experience is basically depleting or rewarding, I believe, is to a large extent determined by the way staff members deal with the emotions stimulated in them by the situations. Whenever we tolerate behavior, we tend to feel depleted because emotions are aroused in us which we keep in check with a large expenditure of energy. On the other hand, if we can use the experience of the arousal of these emotions as an opportunity to come to grips with issues raised and thus gain mastery, we tend to feel replenished.

Disturbed individuals, on the one hand, arouse our emotions more intensely than most people, since their actions and affect are more intensely conflictual and primitive; on the other hand, they are unusually sensitive to our reactions. It is therefore both more difficult and more urgent that those who work with the severely disturbed be able to deal effectively with their own emotional reactions. There is some similarity to the problems of dealing with young children and with those we love most. Both of these groups of people arouse our most primitive and most conflictual emotions, and both groups are most sensitive to us. I say this not to imply that those whom we love most are most disturbed, but to imply that what we learn about ourselves by working with disturbed people can also be useful in other areas of our lives.

So, while a psychoanalytic approach teaches us that we must be very attentive to the words and actions of those whom we treat, it also teaches us that we must be very attentive to our own inner reactions. This principle can be derived also from the practice of psychoanalysis, which requires that an analyst must be analyzed.

In our work we see over and over again the value of knowledge of ourselves in facilitating our relationships with others. We see self-knowledge, first, as an enabling force in removing obstacles to our understanding of others, and second, as a most valuable source of that same understanding of others. At times our own emotions prevent us from understanding another person. Any mental health professional knows how much easier it is to understand other people's children, parents, marriage, than it is to understand one's own. We believe that there is a common human unconscious, that within the depths of our minds lies a common human experience, so that the knowledge of those depths is a rich source of empathic understanding. It is important that we can feel, "There but for the grace of God go I." The implication of this statement is that we are all capable of being like another under the appropriate circumstances. The world of art and literature speaks in support of this conviction. There is a lasting body of art and literature of the world, that speaks across national boundaries and is meaningful even in translation, because there are common human themes that appeal to the common human unconscious throughout the ages and cultures of the world. The universal and continuing popularity of these literary and artistic productions reaffirms our conviction that we can understand each other.

It is the fear of this very truth—that there is a common human core and that we are like each other—that sometimes stands in the way of empathy with disturbed people. When a social worker in a mental hospital told her fellow workers that she had feelings similar to those of one of the patients, the other workers reacted with horror. In their minds, to be able to have feelings like a patient was too dangerously close to being a patient. Similarly, a counselor who worked with a group of very aggressive boys was afraid to admit that she, too, enjoyed watching horror movies, lest she be considered to be as aggressively dangerous as the boys with whom she worked. Her anxiety about this admission prevented her from examining the similarities and differences, so she was not able effectively either to refuse to let them watch such movies or to help them to manage the aggressions stimulated and the tremendous anxiety aroused when she did let them watch such movies.

In our work we find that it is very helpful when the staff is encouraged and supported in admitting to some of their own "unacceptable" reactions. Often the release and comfort afforded enables them to continue some action that has become burdensome, or sort out their priorities as to what they think is most important. For example, there are times when it seems desirable that some members of the staff stay up at night with one or another of their charges. When this is an occasional occurrence it does not present much of a problem; the counselor is usually agreeable to being called, and the loss of sleep seems a small price to pay for the degree of comfort it gives to the child and for the degree to which it solidifies the relationship of trust. However, when it becomes a frequent occurrence, it becomes more problematic. The counselor might feel a bad counselor for not enjoying being awakened in the middle of the night to give sustenance to a miserable child in distress. If the counselor continues to go to the child, often a feeling of resentment is built up which exacerbates the nighttime problem.

There have been occasions when the counselor's freedom (with support and encouragement from other staff members) to express anger at being awakened, and the sympathy evoked from other staff members, have been sufficient to permit the counselor to recognize a wish to continue this practice, which is very beneficial to the child and, though tiring, is beneficial to the counselor in filling a therapeutic role. On other occasions it has become clear that a counselor needs more relief in a realistic way, perhaps to be relieved of some daytime responsibility. In still other situations it has become clear that it is not wise for the counselor to go to the child. When a girl with a history of sleeping in her parents' bedroom would stay awake for hours, we decided that it would be best for the counselors not to stay with her. People were available outside of the dormitory for her, but no one stayed in the room with her. She gradually learned to sleep without the company of an adult. The counselors in effecting this decision needed reassurance that it was for the good of the child, and not because of their complaints of lack of sleep. In all cases, recognizing and accepting the emotional reaction of the staff has been a necessary first step in effective decision making.

Many times and in many ways emotional reactions that are unacceptable to ourselves can interfere with our understanding. In work with children who are severely disturbed or in other ways different from us we frequently have negative reactions, sometimes because their actions are very hard to take or impose something difficult on us, like losing sleep, or being sworn at, and at other times because their actions or attitudes are threatening to us, like dirtiness or blatant sexuality. No matter what the reason, when our emotional reaction is unacceptable to us, it is very important that we recognize and deal with it, so that by inducing distancing and distortion it does not prevent us from being close to our children and understanding their needs.

Because of its importance, in our work we often ask each other about our emotional reaction to a behavior or event. It is interesting how frequently staff members are reluctant to answer this question, afraid that their reaction, unacceptable to themselves, will also be unacceptable to fellow workers. However, despite resistance we persist, and many times when we are having some difficulty in our work, if we can simply manage to discuss with each other our emotional reactions, the difficulties are resolved in a way that seems almost magical. Such was the case when a psychotic boy was tearing his clothes. The counselor closest to him first talked about her reaction to the waste of money involved. We realized that if his tearing his clothes would lead him closer to rehabilitation, it would be money well spent. This recognition helped her to be less tense about the clothes-tearing. She further examined her reaction, relating it to her own feelings about the importance of clothes to her when she was a child and in a situation separated from her parents. That clothes were so emotionally significant to her made it difficult for her to emotionally tolerate seeing the boy tear clothes. After she had this realization, the boy stopped tearing his clothes. We speculated that it was likely that her response to him and his clothes became less fraught with her own emotional issues, and that she was therefore free to be more empathic on a nonverbal level. Since the new message she conveyed, though very powerful, was nonverbal, she was unable to document it, and thus the effect seemed magical.

Though the recognition of emotional responses, as I have said, often leads to resolution of problems, it certainly does not always. In order to know how to deal with our young people we have to do much more. First we have to understand them, and then we have to know how to plan for their therapeutic growth and learning. Empathy is an avenue toward understanding. In our efforts to use self-knowledge in understanding we often try to imagine how we would feel if we were in the shoes of our children. Since it is our conviction that there is much in common in our unconscious, self-knowledge is a significant way of understanding. It has a value deeper than that of understanding from a textbook, because understanding derived from one's own heart conveys to the other person a closeness and acceptance that is at least as valuable as the understanding itself.

In this respect a staff member's own analysis is often a valuable tool. Severely disturbed children often experience the world as though from raw emotions, without protection. Their experiences can be considered akin to the experience of an analysand: having laid aside defenses for the hour, the analysand looks inward at disorganized, primary process, raw emotion, coming from all areas of life, from the earliest years of nonverbal experience to the most recent, most sophisticated experience. Our understanding is that our children have not been able to develop adequate defenses, that their egos are deficient, deficient in processing and organizing their experience and in developing adequate means of coping with life; the way they feel is much like the feeling of the analysand in the most disorganized, distressing periods of analysis.

Fortunately, it is not always necessary to go to these most drastic means to develop empathy. The experience of those with undeveloped egos is also akin to that of children at an early age. One of our consultants in his teaching suggests to the staff that they actually, physically, put themselves in the position of a child to remember how it feels. He has staff members feed each other, with the one being fed having no verbal ability to control the feeder. The staff is usually amazed at the feeling of frustrated helplessness that occurs when one wants to be fed but has a feeder who is out of tune with one's needs. Such techniques are often very useful on the road to understanding. If we talk like the child, walk like the child, hold ourselves like the child, we can begin to feel how it feels to be that child.

This has been a discussion of attitudes—attitudes toward the persons we are trying to help, and attitudes toward ourselves—that derive from a psychoanalytic stance and that we have found helpful in our work with children and adolescents who have difficulty in mastering life. There is much more to be learned, and that we have learned, from explorations in the field of psychoanalysis. Our understanding has been deepened by this accumulated knowledge and theory, and the interpretations expressed in some of my vignettes reflect some of this. However, I want to emphasize the attitudes I have discussed as the sine qua non of psychoanalytically oriented milieu therapy because throughout the years of my work it has been the warmth, acceptance, and respect that we have had for our young people that have been most effective in moving them toward health.

THREE

Discipline
(Does It Have to Hurt?)

It is another misconception of a psychoanalytic approach that if one simply practices the warmth, acceptance, and respect emphasized in the preceding chapter, that no punishments will be necessary. This is perhaps an outgrowth of the knowledge of the value of free expression emanating from the couch, with a disregard of the restriction of the couch and of the well-developed structure of the typical person on it. That is, many well-structured neurotic people have experienced significant personal growth as a result of the uncovering and freeing brought about by their experience in analysis or psychoanalytic therapy. Some people believe that the acceptance and encouragement of free expression of itself will lead to healthy development. This belief disregards the fact that in the typical analytic situation, free expression is encouraged only within a very restrictive situation—that of lying down with physical activity severely limited.

Anyone who has worked with children in any enterprise, be it designated therapeutic, educational, neither or both, knows that the issue of discipline has to be addressed in order for the individual and the social unit to function. The less inner discipline exists, the more carefully and thoroughly does external discipline have to be considered.

In an institution for children, a majority of whom have little inner discipline, and where we do not use drugs, mechanical restraints, or quiet rooms, the question has to arise as to what we do about aggression, noncompliance, and chaotic behavior. In the chapters that have preceded this one, and in some that will follow, I believe that I have addressed that question in a variety of ways which I will later in this chapter review. However, in them I make no mention of what might be called aversive techniques. None of my cast of characters so much as tells a child to "stop it." There was a time in my career that I would have explained the omission by saying that it was not very important how destructive behavior was stopped as long as it was stopped quickly. I was not interested in concentrating on modes of doing so, but rather would concentrate on understanding how to prevent it from occurring in the first place.

Though I still prefer (obviously) to concentrate on this aspect of the problem, I no longer believe that how destructive behavior is stopped is unimportant. I think that not to discuss it would be a serious omission, because aggression, noncompliance, and chaotic behavior do occur even in the best places, with the most sensitive and experienced staff. Some form of constraints have to be used, and how this is done does make a significant impact. I do not address the question easily, because we have reached neither theoretical nor practical clarity about it. I have chosen to discuss the issue even without closure, because not to do so might give the impression that we do not have the problem at all and do not use any aversive methods.

Before discussing aversive techniques, I would like first to review some of the ingredients that go into the development of that internal discipline that is, of course, most desirable. This internal discipline involves both the ability to control oneself and the desire to do so, in line with the expectations and needs of the society of which one is a part. Self-control is, in terms of our theoretical approach, an ego function. Since the ego becomes stronger in its excercise, providing situations wherein children are able to successfully exercise self-control is critical in our efforts to help them develop it. Further, providing those conditions which will increase the likelihood of our youngsters desiring to exercise such control is also critical. These situations and conditions can usefully be considered in the following categories: characteristics of the environment, clarity and consistency of expectation, consistent models for identification, manageable degree of stress conditions, and understanding.

An environment that is clearly ordered physically, temporally, and in its expectations is easily mastered and, therefore, facilitates the development of self-discipline. The early Montessori environment is a good example of this.[1]

When equipment has its place, as in a typical Montessori nursery school, on low reachable shelves that are wide enough for only one piece of equipment at a time, it is almost as easy for a child to put a toy back on its shelf as to leave it on the floor. The value of its not being on the floor to trip on is evident enough so that the discipline of orderliness is fairly easily developed. This is the principle that we try to follow in our arrangement of the School. The purposes of the various spaces are designed to be clear. The temporal organization is designed to be in keeping with the needs and abilities of the students. And the expectations are designed to be both clear and within the capabilities of the students. For example, the distinction between quiet and active times and places has to be readily apparent to students. They will then have the environmental indicator that the class at 9:15 is not a place and time to run around, which will help them carry out the teacher's verbal admonition to stay in their places. In addition, in order for students to be able to conform to this clearly presented expectation, it is important that the time for quiet does not exceed their capability to remain inactive. In a School as small as ours, schedules can be tailored to individual needs to a large, but still limited, degree. The presence of staff members who know the students well provides a flexibility in degree of support and adjustment of expectation that enables the students to be self-disciplined even when the organization of the environment as a whole is not fine-tuned to each one's individual needs. For example, in a class of six the first period of the day might be forty-five minutes devoted to math, because this is the time the children are most alert and most able to concentrate on this kind of abstraction. Within this period the teacher has to make further adjustments because each child may have a different attention span and a different tolerance for seat work. Child A, who can concentrate for not more than ten minutes, alternates ten minutes of math with ten minutes of drawing. Child B, who needs success at the start of the day, is first given problems the nature of which B has already clearly mastered. Child C works steadily at a desk for forty-five minutes, and Child D builds with blocks for forty-five minutes. In this way all of the children conform to the expectation of the math period, which has been designed in keeping with their average capabilities and adjusted to their individual capabilities.

In order to be able to comply with expectations, the individual has to know what the expectations are. Young and fragile people cannot manage rapidly changing expectations, or seriously differing expectations among those most closely responsible for them. It is for this reason that we organize the School so as to facilitate frequent communication among the staff and endeavor to have the School as unified as possible. We meet daily with as many of the staff as possible attending the meetings.

A most striking example of the effectiveness of communication among staff as an approach in developing discipline occurred at a nursery school and day care center. There was a rash of profanity that the director of the program felt was entirely inappropriate for the age group. Efforts to curtail it seemed ineffective. It was felt that there was a disagreement among the staff as to the desirability of permitting such behavior: the nursery school staff thought that the day care staff permitted it. A meeting of the entire staff was called to discuss the issue. It became very quickly apparent that no one thought that it should be permitted. However, it also became apparent that many of the staff were ambivalent about it. Some felt that it really was all right for little children to swear, but since it would embarrass their parents and the center, it was better that they should not. Some felt that it was not all right for little children to swear, but they themselves had as children received such harsh injunctions against it, that they in fact enjoyed the freedom they imagined the children having when they swore. After this general meeting and discussion there was a very marked diminishment of the swearing. Apparently when the teachers were able to clarify their own thinking about the issue of swearing, and to recognize that they all really supported (though for differing reasons) the administration's policy about it, they were able to present a consistent expectation to the children, and little else was necessary. The children knew very clearly what was expected of them and were able to comply.

This example demonstrates that the need for consistency is both interindividual and intraindividual. The teachers had to be in agreement—it could not be o.k. for a child to swear in front of teacher A and not o.k. to swear in front of teacher B. To manage this variety of behavior takes greater inner integration than a nursery school child has usually achieved, especially if there is an inconsistency within the administration. The teachers also had to be internally consistent. Children who heard a teacher telling them to stop swearing, but sensed the teacher's enjoyment of the swearing, might have had a hard time responding only to what the teacher was saying.

This example also illustrates the extent to which children can distinguish different social entities. It was not important to involve parents in this issue, though it was important to involve all staff. It is likely that the behavior in question was related to appropriate school behavior in the view of the children, rather than to a more general appropriateness. Children who are psychologically ready for an ordinary school environment are able to tolerate differences in expectations from different social groups. Younger and more fragile children are not able to do so.

For normal children this example would indicate that the necessary consistency is that of the intraindividual consistency and of the interindividual consistency of the social group. That is, adults in the same school, the same recreational group, or the same family should strive for a consistency of expectation.

In our efforts to help develop internal discipline in children and adolescents, the issue of consistency with the administration (the principal, the director, the boss, the ultimate authority, the super-ego figure) is an important one. In order for the expectations to be consistent and clear, the staff has to support the expectations of the administration. The issue becomes very difficult if the staff does not agree with the administration's expectations. For this reason I tried to have no rules, except that no one be allowed to hurt anyone (self included). Instruction to new counselors were simply to keep the children safe and try to help them have a good time. New teachers were to try to get to know their students' learning levels and interests. Any way of doing things that we had developed would be open to question, and I usually would tell people that if they didn't believe something was right they shouldn't do it; if they didn't understand a practice, they should follow it on good faith and question it as soon as possible. Our frequent meetings were for the purpose of being able to have a meeting of minds so that our approach to our students could be consistent.

This ideal of consensus is, of course, only an ideal; and we have come to have, if not rules, very clear standards and mores. In reality, even if it were possible to predict every issue that would come up, and even if there were time in this life to discuss every issue, it is unimaginable that even two people could agree on everything. Nonetheless, it is important to maintain the ideal since it increases the possibility that the most important issues to any individual will be discussed and, if not agreed upon, at least understood in such a way that they could be clearly presented. Then, if an administrator takes an action which both teacher and student dislike, a teacher could say (in, of course, more natural wording) to a complaining student, "I don't like it either but the principal's reasons for doing so were . . . ; I explained that there were the following reasons for not doing so: . . . Since the decision, with which I do not agree, was made in good faith for what our principal believed to be the best interest of us all, I think we should follow it in good faith."

Such a statement presupposes a mutual agreement on some basic issues relating to the idea of what is good for the students and the institution, as well as mutual respect. If these exist, it is possible for there to be disagreement about many issues, but for mutual support to continue. A clear statement of disagreement, with reasons for it and reasons for continued support, is much more facilitating of the development of discipline than a false or blind statement of agreement.

When both teacher and student feel that they can be heard, the development of discipline is encouraged. When all who are involved feel that they are parties to the development and maintenance of the expectations of the environment, they are more likely to support them. Thus it is important that students feel that they can tell the teacher or principal when they think that an action is inconsistent with the basic philosophy of the institution or does them personal damage. In order for them to be able to do this, the philosophy of the institution has to be clear to them. As Director of the School I would try to facilitate this understanding in a variety of ways. I would explain the School to every child who came, and whenever possible explain my actions in terms of the School's philosophy. I would meet with all of the children together once a week and talk to them together on significant occasions (holidays, the arrival of a new child, graduation, and any time something happened that affected the entire School). When I did so I would explain the occasion in terms of the School's general philosophy. I would invite questions and comments. When students reach the age of fourteen they are voluntary members of the School's community and, therefore, if they do not agree with the philosophy of the School they are free to leave. Their staying at the School commits them, then, to upholding the philosophy. This commitment can be effective if they feel that they are able also to influence it. In our efforts to achieve consistency, we thus engage the students in the process of clarification and support.

Students in varying degree identify with the adults around them. By identification I am now simply referring to the phenomenon of acting like another person. It is difficult to determine with whom a young person will identify and to what degree that identification will occur. However, we do know that it is a very common phenomenon. It behooves us then to consider ourselves as we present ourselves in relation to the issue of discipline. Our students know that we believe discipline to be important. Some of our more sophisticated wiseacres, upon discovering that a staff member does not have certain reports in on time, have righteously asked how the staff member could possibly expect a student to have homework done on time (no matter if the teacher was late because of filling in on an emergency). This kind of behavior is, of course, a nuisance but it can lead to a serious discussion of the important issue. What is seriously to be considered is the real identification that takes place when a staff member has an attitude of noncompliance: if the staff member, for example, does not really make a serious effort to have things done in a timely fashion. The student is then as likely to identify with this attitude as to respond to a teacher's requests for timeliness in homework.

Everyone tends to function better when not under undue stress. This better functioning includes those functions related to discipline. One can better control one's negative impulses and proceed systematically toward one's goals when one is not stressed. Under conditions of stress I include excessively distressing emotion, anxiety, and temptation. The person with aggressive tendencies is less likely to act on them when not angry, feeling frustrated, or otherwise upset. The person with delinquent tendencies is less likely to steal when there is no temptation.

Therefore, we try to arrange the environment so as to reduce the available temptations. All money is locked up, as are all potentially dangerous items. Anything that is broken is removed and repaired as quickly as possible. We in general try to reduce as much as possible the conditions that might lead to the stimulation of anger or acute anxiety. In our planning of activities, for example, we are very careful about the issue of competition. We at times redesign athletic games so as to soften the competitive edge. All of our efforts that make the world more manageable for our students help them to be more disciplined.

Understanding the students, both individually and in general, is, of course, prerequisite to creating an environment that enables them to be as disciplined as possible. In prior chapters I have presented examples of how a staff member's understanding in particular instances enabled a child who had been acting undisciplined to become disciplined by himself. The little boy who was running about the house could settle down and go to sleep when we listened to him and made a "tornados go that way" sign. The teenager who had been obscene and loud became apologetic and decent when we recognized that he had had reason to be upset.

This has been a brief review of some of the components significant in the development of a disciplined person. Underlying all of them is a basic component of trust. As the teenager earlier referred to said to me in explaining his compliance to me but not to his counselors, "I will do what you or Dr. B. tell me even when I don't agree because I think you have my best interest at heart."

When there is a breakdown in discipline, it is most important to consider what the cause of it might be and to respond in

DISCIPLINE (DOES IT HAVE TO HURT?)

those terms. Much of the time, increased understanding leads to measures that will reduce stress (either by external changes or attention to internal issues), clarify expectations, and otherwise lead to means of developing discipline. However, situations do occur when aggression, noncompliance, and chaotic behavior seem to require action that I characterize as aversive.

There is, I believe, an important distinction to be made in regard to discipline in general and self-control in particular. This is the distinction between the ability to be self-disciplined and the desire to be so. In dealing with disciplinary issues, it is important to be able to distinguish which is predominant: that is, whether a person is acting in a destructive manner as a result of being unable to do otherwise, or as a result of not wishing to do otherwise.

When I was about to take on the position of Director of the School, a fairly large teenager asked me what I would do if he hit me. I didn't answer the question because I didn't know what the answer would be. I probably said, "I don't know." At that point, I did not know the boy well enough to know whether he was worried about my ability (since I am a relatively small woman, obviously weaker than he) to contain his unmanageable (to him) aggression, or whether he was assessing if I was an administrator smart enough to contend with his intense but manageable (to him) aggression. In retrospect my naive but honest answer was probably the appropriate one. This young man had the ability to control his aggression, but not always the desire to do so. A few months ealier another teenager had been expelled for hitting the man who was the Director of the School at that time. It is fairly likely that the boy who approached me with the question was considering whether or not hitting me would be a way out for him, since he was very ambivalent about staying at the School. In reconsidering the incident, at times I thought that I should have asked, "Why would you want to hit me?" I had no intention of doing anything that would make him angry enough at me to hit me. Asking the question would have let him know that I was interested in his anger and might have helped me to understand how to reduce it.

To a significant extent, understanding others enables one to know what is likely to make them act in a destructive or chaotic fashion. We try to act in ways so as not to induce such behavior. However, it is at times necessary to act in a way that will make another person angry. A child who cannot tolerate failure still has to be told that a wrong solution to an addition problem is wrong. We might try to present the information in as supportive a manner as possible, but the message has to be given even if it precipitates the tearing up of the book. When I do anything vis-à-vis a child that I believe is likely to make so much anger that I might be in danger of attack, I make sure that I am in a position to control the child physically with relative ease, or if it is a child that I cannot myself control physically I always am sure that there are enough people nearby who are obviously capable of doing so.

When a child is in a tantrum I just make sure that there is no one close enough to be hurt, and that nothing very valuable or irreplaceable is around. We often hold a child who is attacking self or others to make sure that no damage is done to a person. We try to release the hold as soon as possible so that the child can begin to exercise self-control. Usually, after the tantrum is over, the child is willing enough to settle down; frequently the child will gladly do some kind of retributive work. In these tantrums, the child usually has the desire for self-control but not the ability to exert it and, therefore, basically perceives the holding and containment as support. Afterwards, doing something to make up for the destruction helps the child to recapture a sense of mastery and self-esteem.

When a child is in a chaotic state, in my experience the presence of a trusted person can serve as an integrative focus that helps the child become more contained. I have been able to help a schizophrenic young woman stop pacing and violently slamming things around, by having her look at me. It seems that when she would look at me, and would see that I was neither angry nor disorganized, she would be able to experience the positive aspects of our relationship and thereby reintegrate herself. For some children a very strong show of power achieves similar results. A child lying screaming on the floor of the dining room will often be able to get up and calmly walk out of the room when three big men stand by, and one suggests that either the child walk out self-propelled or be carried out by them.

At the School, it was customary procedure for me to be called in to settle a chaotic or destructive situation. A substantial part of the time my presence was settling. I believe that this was partly because of the students' recognition of the power I wielded (I could, for example, call in extra people to impose my will or expel children) and partly because of the nature of my relationship with them when it was one of trust that I was acting in their best interest and would be fair to them. For the more severely disturbed children in particular, I could sometimes be effective in this way because I represented a constant and dependable person.

It is very important that children with weak egos are able to feel that they can be controlled by someone else. They otherwise feel at the mercy of their chaotic impulses. Even though they protest, they are very much relieved when they find that someone else can control them and prevent them from acting out their inner chaos. As Erikson has elaborated throughout his discussion of mutuality in the stages of psychosocial development, the appropriate balance is critical.[2] So, though it is necessary for the child to feel that others can be in control, it is at the same time important that this not be overcontrol. It is our belief that children's success in reestablishing integration strengthens their ability to control themselves. We, therefore, prefer to exert as little external constraint as possible so as to facilitate this development. If the external control is exerted in excessive amounts, or on inappropriate occasions, then the child will have the feeling of helplessness.

This kind of external control is not usually aversive and, if a child is at all rational, is not experienced as punitive. There is another kind of reaction to destructive behavior that seems also to help develop discipline and is not usually experienced as punitive by the child who really wants to become disciplined. This is what can be called restitutive action. That is, a person who has engaged in destructive behavior does something to make amends for the destruction. A child who marks up a wall, washes it; a child who tears up a book, repairs it; a child who breaks a window, pays for it. There are some children who view even this as punishment, but there are many other children who spontaneously try to make restitution, and many who when assigned such tasks feel relieved and are eager to make amends.

All of the discussion so far still does not take into account all aspects of the disciplinary process, and there are situations that seem to call for action that in common parlance would be called punishment. Though I have never accepted whole-heartedly the maxim "spare the rod and spoil the child," there was a time when I thought that the best way to deal with those situations requiring aversive or punitive action was with a good hard smack on the shoulder. (The face is too humiliating, and the backside is too close to the erotic zone.) The first time such a situation arose with my own son was when he was a toddler and had cheerfully taken his little wooden hammer and broken a window. My serious "no-no" and removal of the hammer seemed to make no impact on his cheerfulness, and it seemed that there was no way to make clear to him that he was not to break windows, except by a smack. One of our psycho-analytic consultants reported to me that his nonviolent disciplinary approach broke down when his youngster ran out into the street. I recall that at the time of the hammer incident, I was not angry at my boy, but only desperate to impress upon him an important point; I believe my colleague had similar feelings. I do not mean to imply that there was no other way, only that we could think of no other way. Fortunately, there were not many other occasions when I found myself in that position with my son, and, according to his report, the few incidents of physically punitive disciplinary measures that he remembers had little significance to him.

There is a significant necessity for strong measures in order to make a position clear in an institution having many staff members and dealing with youngsters who do not easily per-ceive things accurately. I have earlier discussed the impor-tance of interstaff consistency. When for a certain kind of be-havior there is a clear and obvious punishment that is clearly and consistently administered, there is little likelihood of mis-understanding, among the staff or children, that the behavior is unacceptable. Frequently members of the staff have mis-takenly believed that I condoned a certain kind of behavior, for example, swearing and speaking disrespectfully to a staff member, of which I actually disapprove strongly. If I refrain from criticizing a girl swearing at me during a tantrum and in later staff discussion concentrate on trying to understand the behavior, it might lead to the staff's believing that it is o.k. for children to swear and be disrespectful routinely, without any particular provocation. In the ideal I would be able to have a thorough discussion of every such incident. Then all staff would clearly understand that I did not criticize because the child in question knew very well my position on swearing and disrespect, but in that particular situation could not conform. They would know that my efforts had been to understand and strengthen her so that she would be able to act on what she knew, and be more able not to swear or be disrespectful in general. However, since the ideal can only seldom be attained, and since too much destructive behavior can destroy the fabric of any society, it is important to have ways, which may at times be aversive and punitive, that convey very clear messages throughout an institution as to what is acceptable and what is not.

Another area where we have found aversive measures to be indicated is in regard to the destructive acting out of some youngsters who basically believe they should not be destructive, but are either so angry at the time that they do not care, or simply get more relief from the acting out than pleasure from the control of it. When they are small enough, such children can be held by the hand to be contained. It is much more problematic when they are too big and strong for this. In our experience a "good smack" has contained them. The more disorganized of these youngsters often claim child abuse and complain about the hurtfulness of such a smack, but they seem much better integrated and relieved immediately after the smack. One better-organized early teenager reported afterwards that he felt that it was important and helpful that this was done. When his acting out occurred, he was in a very difficult period: he had just entered puberty, and a most significant counselor had just left. He had begun acting out in a way that was unusual for him, running off the grounds, spitting at staff members, and the like. With the punishment, the gross acting out stopped, and he was very much relieved. For this kind of child, punishment also seems to serve the purpose of alleviating guilt and thereby lessens the need for further acting out, or engagement in self-punitive measures.

Most difficult to contend with is the youngster who has not yet developed a significantly strong alliance with the staff and has a tendency toward destructive, disobedient, or chaotic action. There is a degree to which such children will engage in this kind of action because it is an outlet for the pressure of their generalized (or specific) anger and because there is no deterrent. Since they have little or no attachment, there is no inner deterrent, and there is no positive force or motive strong enough to balance the relief experienced by the discharge. A punitive consequence can sometimes provide a deterrent. But if the consequence is considered inequitable to the youngster, it is likely to be alienating. It then lessens the likelihood of the development of positive attachments and identification that will lead to conscience and to discipline in the positive sense.

The child who is already on the side of self-control is likely to see a punitive consequence for destructive action as just, much more readily than the child who is not yet on the side of self-control. For this reason, the students at the School have accepted that I "go easy on a kid" for the first year or so. That is, all of the students know that newcomers can get away with a lot that a senior person cannot, because they need time to develop attachments to the School and to understand that there is value and good reason to behave.

Ideally, then, no punitive action should be taken until identification and relationships are established, so that the punishment is perceived as just and on the side of development of the kind of discipline that is the child's own. (I do not mean to imply that destructive behavior should not be contained or criticized; this statement refers only to aversive, punitive, action.) However this ideal for some children is difficult to realize because the nature of their destructive acts make it necessary for aversive measures to be imposed before they have been able to develop the positive identifications and relationships that help them to view such measures as supportive. This necessity is sometimes a result of the intensity of the behavior and sometimes a result of the difficulty in developing relationships.

There is a need for protection of others both from being hurt and from anxiety about being hurt. When a child is acting out destructively, other staff members and students often have hostile, negative reactions. These, of course, can (and should) be dealt with in terms of the particular significance to each individual. For example, a student who loudly complains about another student's aggressive behavior, on closer analysis might be found to be getting vicarious pleasure from the acting out of that aggressive behavior and sometimes even will have provoked it in the acting-out individual. While this aspect is of great importance to deal with, it is also of great importance that undue anxiety not be created and that the children see that they will be protected from the acting out of others.

Staff, too, need both help in dealing with their reactions and security that they will be protected. If a staff member is actually hurt, a reaction of anger might be appropriate and need not be analyzed as related to anything other than the hurt. A staff member sometimes needs help in accepting the value of directly expressing that anger to the offender. Frequently staff members who are not directly involved with the disruptive youngster become angry; anger at the child who is acting out almost seems to become a receptacle into which many dissatisfactions can be funneled. These issues ideally should be dealt with in supervision and staff meetings. However, even with the best efforts, the consequences of these feelings are sometimes directed to the acting-out child.

A punitive action can be helpful in addressing at least two aspects of the problem of staff's and children's reactions to a child who is destructive and disruptive. Most people feel, rationally or not, that when the offender is punished they are protected. Therefore, a punishment reduces the anxiety among those affiliated with an aggressive person. In addition, it satisfies some of the anger that is, rationally or not, aroused by the child. A punitive action can temporarily reduce this generalized anger and is better than the effects of a rejecting attitude.

It may be that in some theoretical heaven children can be raised without a containment or punishment system; perhaps in that theoretical heaven even severely emotionally disturbed children and adolescents can live and go to school together without a containment or punishment system. I do not believe that it is possible here on earth. Whatever system is used, I believe that it is very important that it be flexible, so that its balance can be adjusted as needed to be perceived as supportive rather than alienating, and so that it can yield maintenance of control to the internal system as soon as possible.

I cannot answer the question of what the ideal system should be. All I can do is present some of our experience and reflect on it. For several years, I thought that the best system was to use a strong and careful hit. It was quick and clear, and I was the only one authorized to administer it. The staff could hit in self-defense; though we were aware that at times one can lose one's temper, there was otherwise no condoning of the staff's hitting. I felt that my being the only one to hit would insure some distance and would reduce the likelihood of the action's being taken out of anger. I had not been involved with the action of the student that led to the punishment, but was being called in to settle the misbehavior. Furthermore, being the most experienced person on the staff, I believed (perhaps somewhat arrogantly) that I had the best possibility of awareness of my motivations. When I began to feel that my hits were for some students a bit of a joke, given the gentleness of my most vigorous assault, I sometimes had a male staff member administer the smacks under my supervision.

There were times, as I have suggested, that this approach accomplished its purpose with no apparent ill effects. But gradually some ill effects began to be apparent to me. Of these, there were four varieties: (1) we became the abusers of abused children; (2) children who had aggressive tendencies identified with this aspect of our approach; (3) we became actors in unconscious sexual-sado-masochistic fantasies; and (4) we sent out negative messages that we were not aware of.

(1) Those of our children who had been abused simply did not care about any kind of punishment because no matter what we did, it did not compare with what they had suffered. To have any effect we would have to become more and more punitive. We found that punishment was extremely difficult to manage, because a child who has been abused easily manages to arouse the desire to be abusive in even the most benign

caretakers. Actually hitting the child makes the arousal even stronger. Though for these children any kind of punishment is generally ineffective, physical punishment seems worst as it makes the present world much the same as the past in its abusiveness.

(2) Since our closeness to our students encourages the formation of identifications, we behave in a fashion that is absolutely contradictory when we instruct them not to hit, but do so ourselves. It is a much more significant issue to those who have themselves the tendency to be aggressive, since they are much more likely to identify with it. After I announced that we had adopted a policy of absolutely no hitting of students, our adolescent boys reported that there was a marked decrease in the hitting of each other that had been going on when there were no staff members present.

(3) I was surprised, in the process of changing our policy, to find that I had not been as astute in my self-knowledge as I had imagined. This revelation was particularly cogent around a youngster who had masochistic fantasies and did not object to my hitting him. I was humbled to realize suddenly that I had been making myself a partner to his disturbed fantasies.

(4) In the area of unknown messages, I include my experience with an adolescent girl suffering from pervasive developmental disorder. I had been using hitting to contain her nightime chaos. It had been effective in enabling her to settle down and sleep. I did not know just what I was going to substitute, but I decided to stop smacking her. As soon as I did so, her chaotic behavior lessened dramatically. I cannot explain this.

With the initiation of a policy of no hitting, the need for a containment and punishment system did not disappear. I still believe that my "good hard hit on the arm" was preferable and less punitive than isolation rooms, drugs, or restraints, so we have not been willing to turn to those methods. The other methods that we have thought of until now have been neither entirely satisfactory nor entirely unsatisfactory. We therefore continue to use some combination of them all.

Perhaps the most satisfactory method is an extension of what I have already referred to as restitutive activity. We assign the student a moderately unpleasant task which benefits the commonweal. A problem with this approach for students not on the side of discipline development is that it is difficult to make them do such tasks without a stronger punitive back-up. What do we do if a student refuses to sweep the floor? Another problem is that it often takes a good deal of ingenuity to find appropriate tasks, and they often require staff supervision. For example, cleaning is an appropriate restitutive activity, since a children's institution rarely has enough regular staff to do all the cleaning that might be desirable, few children really like to clean, and it is a real contribution to the general well-being. However, most children need to be taught how to clean and supervised in order for the cleaning to be effective. Though restitution by cleaning makes for a very good and desirable experience in terms of the student's growth, the staff supervisory time might not be available.

Another problem that arises with restitutive activity is that some students enjoy it. In itself this does not detract from its value as a containment measure, since by doing an enjoyable, constructive activity that contributes to the good of society, the student feels better and more identified with the society. At the same time there is a kind of discomfort amongst staff and other students at the idea that a child gets to do something enjoyable as a result of a misdemeanor.

Yet another drawback to this mode is that the activities so used become tainted. For example, we might use snow-shoveling as a restitutive activity. There are a number of youngsters who, when they see snow on a weekend or holiday, might volunteer to clear the walks and consider it to be a privilege when they are permitted to do so. However, if during the previous snowfall some students were assigned to shovel the walks as a consequence of destructive behavior, the good citizens might be reluctant to volunteer their services.

I have been hesitant to withdraw privileges as a consequence of destructive or disruptive behavior. Usually when we grant a privilege to an individual, for example, when we allow a student to go to an outside library to do research for a report, it is because we believe that the privilege granted will be growth-inducing. This kind of privilege requires the exercise of the student's most highly integrated, mature behavior. To take away the experience might reduce the number of opportunities when this kind of behavior is demanded in a way in which the student wishes to comply. Similarly, taking away recess time for some children is counterproductive. This is especially the case with children who have a great need for physical discharge. The curtailment of assigned time for such discharge makes it much harder for them to contain themselves.

Restrictions on such activities as listening to music or watching television do not seem to have negative side effects. The only problem in this kind of punitive action is that of supervision in our setting. Since the group generally engages in activities together, when one member is not able to watch television or listen to music, extra supervision has to be provided for that child. One relatively minor problem with restricting television or music is that in a subtle way, it gives more value to those activities than we would like.

We have used allowance restriction as a punitive mode; it has the advantage of being fairly visible, clear, and not overly harsh. All of our students get a weekly allowance, which they are free to spend on anything they want. A reduction in allowance does not eliminate food treats or entertainment, because snacks and outings are generally provided. Nor does it eliminate toys, books, or other such items, since students receive ample presents on Christmas, other holidays, and their birthdays. Thus the mode is not depriving nor excessively punitive. The amount of allowance lost is related to the amount and seriousness of the transgression. (We use the word "transgression" for the punishable act because it means a crossing of a boundary, rather than "evil," which other terms imply.)

In keeping with our idea that students are members of the community by common consent, it has been suggested that disruptive behavior be dealt with by the community in group meetings. Though I have found that the impact of other students is of inestimable importance, to make use of it at a group meeting is exceedingly difficult. In order for a meeting of severely disturbed youngsters to be a positive experience, their collective health has to be drawn out and emphasized so that healthful striving can be the dominant tone of the meeting. Mutual anxieties and aggressive tendencies are very easily stimulated and even acted upon in a group meeting. Therefore, when an issue of a member's aggression is raised, these tendencies are stimulated, together with related anxieties. As a result the offending youngster might easily be shamed in an open discussion or possibly supported in the offense.

There is ultimately the spoken or unspoken threat of expulsion, if a youngster is basically not conforming to the expectations of the institution. It has been in almost all cases an effective tool. However, it seems appropriate to use it only for extreme violations; much of what takes place that requires attention does not seem to warrant the threat of expulsion. We have at times suspended a youngster in extreme situations. Suspension presents major problems. The students' justifiable criticism of this technique is, "How can you help a kid who isn't here?" Suspension interrupts and may seriously impede the therapeutic process. It also requires significant cooperation on the part of the parents, who need information and support in order to know how to deal with the child appropriately in this critical situation.

I cannot omit from this account my personal style. Though I am most of the time a slow-moving, soft-spoken person, when one of "my kids" has done something that I consider wrong— nasty or destructive—I have usually yelled and screamed. For many, anticipation of being yelled at has been a very effective deterrent to unacceptable behavior. For those who valued my approval, I wouldn't even have to raise my voice. One youngster told me, "You yell more quietly than anyone I know."

FOUR

A Place to Learn

The principles so far discussed pervade the dormitory and classroom environment. They are principles that I believe can be useful in the construction of any educative enterprise. In this chapter I will describe further how we try to effect these and other principles in the classrooms of the School. Much of what we do, of course, is pragmatic and probably based on our prejudices, which will no doubt be included in this exposition as much as our principles.

I will be omitting any discussion of cognitive development, many aspects of curriculum development, approaches to subject matter organization, as well as many other important areas. We do not consider them less important, but they are not my particular areas of expertise. Our teachers come with training and experience in these areas; they share their experience with each other, and we encourage their acquisition of further knowledge and training. In other words, other aspects are very much a part of our enterprise.

The classroom is an integral part of the therapeutic milieu, not only because our children need continuous understanding support, but also because the learning that takes place is itself therapeutic. Learning strengthens the ego's functioning in such areas as perception, motility, and self-control and provides it with the means of better meeting its tasks. The more knowledge one has of the world, the better one is able to master it. Psychoanalytic insights contribute not only to our understanding of what might stand in the way of learning, but also to our understanding of how learning might take place. Underlying all of our educational considerations are the following questions: (1) What are the emotional preconditions of learning? (We know that children must have certain cognitive abilities and have reached certain cognitive levels to master particular tasks. Is it not also likely that they must have certain emotional abilities and have reached certain levels of emotional integration in order to achieve mastery of particular tasks?) (2) What are the emotional facilitators of learning? (3) What are the emotional impediments to learning? (4) What kind of learning can contribute to the emotional well-being of the child? What is to follow does not reflect definite answers to these questions, but is rather our attempt to consider each question as related to a situation and to work out as good an answer as we can.

Just as the physical and human environments are both part of the therapeutic milieu of the School as a whole, they are similarly part of the therapeutic milieu of its educative component. This chapter concentrates on the physical environment, including curriculum considerations, and the next chapter, on the human environment.

There are five classrooms at the School; six or seven students are in each class. (These add up to fewer than our total enrollment because at any given time several students are usually attending classes outside of the School, at the University of Chicago Laboratory School, another local high school, the college of the University of Chicago, or another local college.) The students are with the same teacher all day, usually for several years, so that the teacher has time to develop an understanding of each student that is facilitating of the relationship and of effective teaching.

Primarily as a result of our emphasis on maintaining the consistency of relationships, the student composition of the classrooms is heterogeneous. Our population is relatively small, with a relatively broad range of ages, grade levels, and types of disturbance, so that any kind of homogeneity is logistically difficult to achieve. The number of graduations in any given year is also inconsistent; graduates most likely come from several different classrooms. When a new student comes to the School, the decision as to which classroom that child will go to is influenced as much by emotional and psychological compatibility with the other students in the class as it is by the academic level at which the child is functioning. The decision to accept a child is also dependent on the composition of the classrooms where openings exist, in terms of the compatibility of the applicant.

Though the classrooms are separate and unique entities, they are also very clearly a part of the whole. All the classes meet together in one of our large common rooms (the auditorium or the playroom) at 9:00 o'clock and at 3:00 o'clock, at the beginning and end of the class day. All classes eat the same food in the same dining room at the same time. The physical eduation program and the recess program are planned together so that the classes mix in a variety of ways for both structured and unstructured physical activities. In addition there are usually some special classes that are composed of age-homogeneous groups. All these arrangements serve the purpose of conveying a feeling of unity. They give the students opportunities to interact with students from other classes and to relate to other teachers.

The classrooms are in a building that was once the schoolhouse of the Universalist Church. The church's nave is now our auditorium. This building is connected to the dormitory building by a lovely corridor, lined with brick and colored-glass brick, and with wooden lockers having heraldic shields as decoration. We reconstructed the interior of the classroom building so that each classroom would be of similar size. Each has a different ambiance built in, achieved by different textures on the floor and walls (tile and shiny wallpaper in one, dark wood floor and walls in another, light wood floor and straw walls in a third). Though the real ambiance is provided by the nature of the teacher, we wanted the classrooms themselves to make it apparent that the school considers each teacher and class different and unique. We also did not want the individual attractiveness of a classroom to depend on the chance decorating talents of the individual teacher.

The classrooms were designed to be large enough to have three areas. One area contains the students' and teacher's desks, a second has tables and chairs for group work, and a third has comfortable seating. These areas make clear the availability of three different kinds of activities. Though our teachers are rarely at their desks, over years of experimenting with different arrangements, we realized that the students

consider the teacher's desk important, perhaps as an indication of a consistent presence and authority. It is also important
for each student to have a desk, though how much time is
spent at it varies from student to student. Each student has, of
course, books, and there is much additional educational material available in the classroom. Whether the walls are deco-
rated with students' individual and group productions depends on the propensities of the teacher and students. In the
largest classroom, projects from years past continue to deco-
rate the walls.

As part of the reconstruction project, washrooms were built
adjacent to four of the five classrooms. (We did this as a partial
solution to the problem of unauthorized meetings.) Some students are embarrassed by this closeness, while for some it is a
reassuring advantage. When a youngster is beset by anxiety,
as are most of those in our care, having an adult near enough
to be heard provides an atmosphere of safety. For some of
those who are embarrassed, the proximity of the washrooms is
an impetus for discussion and provides an opportunity to
work through important issues related to their inability to accept themselves, their body processes or products. However,
for some the embarrassment is a reflection of a phase-appro-
priate desire for privacy that we find ways to respect.

The smallness of the classes, the consistency and continuity
of the relationship of the teacher and student, and the teacher's involvement in the treatment consultation and planning
for each student are all means of insuring the teacher's understanding of the psyche of the individual child, and, thereby, of
insuring the teacher's understanding of what, when, and how
best to teach that child.

Just as the classroom areas are clearly divided and deline-
ated as to function, so is the day divided and organized. Both
structures are there to support, not to impose. The structure is
decided upon based on our knowledge of the needs and abilities of our students, and our insistence on adherence to the
structure is dependent on the developmental level and
strengths of each student. The very existence of these clearly
organized entities in space and time helps the child with a frail
ego to function, even when not absolutely able to adhere to the
organization. Similarly, the consistent presence of an adult

helps the child to exercise self-control, because of the knowledge that both understanding and external control are immediately available. The consistent presentation of learning opportunities, whether the child takes advantage of them or not,
provides further continuing stimulation to growth.

One of the first problems to be addressed every day is that
of transition. Some teachers have their own opening cere-
monies, which have been effective in helping students master
the transition from dormitory to class, with the change in
structure and expectation that it implies. One teacher would
have on each child's desk a little piece of a favorite candy and a
small task that the child could do alone. In this way the child
could start the day by not having to give up the comforts of a
less demanding time entirely and by having a successful learning experience. Another teacher always had a little talk with
her students, in which she briefly went over significant events
that might be on her students' minds (things that were going
on at the School, like a staff member's leaving or a child's
outburst, or in the community, like a presidential election or a
storm), with some comment directed at helping the students
to master anxiety related to the events. She would then review
the expected events of the class day. This teacher's style was
rather formal; her little talk conveyed to her students that
though she expected them to "go on with the show," she had
compassion and concern for what might be troubling them.

At the beginning of the school day it is very helpful for the
teacher to gain a sense of the mood of each child. A discussion
of what has happened since the previous meeting is not usually a good method, since such discussions are likely to evoke
the feelings of any disruption (or pleasure) that has occurred
outside of class; dealing with these feelings distracts from the
educational enterprise. Those successful teachers who do not
have a more or less traditional way, as the two described above
do, usually focus on evoking positive anticipation of a learning
experience by first presenting a learning task at which the child
is likely to succeed. As issues come up, the teacher is sensitive
to the need for discussing things that might be pressing on the
child's mind and interfering with attention to the task.

While it is important that the first task of the day be one at
which the child is likely to succeed, it is also important that the

first period of the day be devoted to those tasks requiring the most concentration, since children usually have the most energy at the beginning of the day. Frequently math is the first subject, and reading or history the second. The arts, free reading, and elective subjects are usually at the end of the day, as they tend to require less intense concentration and frequently capture the child's interest more easily. The length of the periods is not uniform, since it is determined by the amount of time a child is able to concentrate.

The morning hours are divided by a midmorning exercise period. We have found that a sensitively administered physical education program contributes significantly to our children's feeling of mastery and competence. Though it is especially difficult for many of our youngsters to engage in physical activity because of their anxieties about the integrity of their bodies, physical injury, and competition, it is especially important and enriching for them when they are able to cope with those anxieties enough to have success in physical mastery. Activities and games have to be selected to match their particular capabilities and interests, and rules often have to be modified so that, for example, competitive strivings do not become overwhelming. Depending on the individual need, we might simply encourage one youngster to participate, while we might insist that another do so. We pay special attention to anxieties about injury and will, for example, stop a game when someone is injured to review exactly how the injury happened and how it might have been prevented. This is done to help give the students a sense of mastery over what happens to them, by helping them realize that injuries do not occur because their bodies are defective or because they are being punished.

The class eats together with its teacher in the common dining room. The period after lunch is frequently a difficult one, as it necessitates another transition. The general relaxation that is natural and desirable immediately after eating is accommodated by having a free period. The problem of how to provide this freedom without its escalating into chaos is one that different teachers have successfully addressed in different ways. One teacher severely limited freedom of choice to more or less sedentary pursuits, such as table games, conversation, reading, and drawing. Another, more athletically inclined teacher engaged his class in such vigorous sport that they were physically exhausted by the end of the period and ready for mental exercise. At one time the group of teachers got together and offered the students a choice of sedentary or sports activities, with the classes intermingled. In this way appropriate supervision could be provided and there could be greater freedom of choice.

By the end of the day, both students and teacher are usually quite tired. The teacher, nonetheless, tries to close with some unifying activity. A number of teachers find reading a story at the end of the day a successful practice, since everyone can have the same experience, with little expected from the students. Most teachers enjoy reading to their students, and even older students often enjoy being read to. Putting everything back in order gives a feeling of coherence to the day and a feeling of readiness for the next day.

In determining the curriculum, which I here define as the deliberate choice of what we teach, we of course try to take full advantage of knowledge accumulated in all disciplines. My discussion here is limited to those aspects of the choice that can and should be influenced by knowledge of the psyche, particularly that derived from psychoanalytic ego psychological theory. This knowledge can contribute to our wisdom as we decide upon, first, the nature of the learning experience that is appropriate for a particular child or group of children and, second, the particular subject matter that should be included in that learning experience. In regard to the first issue, for many of our students the most important learning experiences are of a nature that most children in regular schools have already mastered. For example, a school-phobic child has to learn to trust the classroom environment in order to begin to be able to do any formal learning in school. Another child might first have to learn the acceptability of body processes, and another child might have to learn that it is safe to find things out.

In regard to the second issue, choice of subject matter, the particular topics addressed in the educational material can themselves facilitate learning. For example, a child who was fascinated by weather learned to read from weather-related words presented by his teacher. This unusual choice of beginning words facilitated his learning to read, while it enhanced his ability to predict significant outcomes.

For both of these issues, the nature of the appropriate learning and of the subject matter for it, the theory that I have briefly outlined in chapter I provides guidance, in terms of the individual and also in terms of some general principles that are pertinent to children at particular stages of development. Guided by the theory, we can speculate more wisely as to what kind of learning experiences are psychologically appropriate for a particular child and what kind of topics are likely to attract emotional investment. Further, guided by the theory, we can also speculate more wisely as to what kind of learning experiences are psychologically appropriate for students at a particular stage of development and what kind of topics are likely to attract emotional investment.

Though our students are by no means at a uniform level of development, there are some characteristics that they have in common, which lead us to provide some rather uniform conditions. They all tend to come to us in a state of stress, anxiety, lack of trust, and diminished interest in the world. In the classroom we, therefore, provide an atmosphere of reduced stress, of meeting their needs, and of attracting them to the surrounding world.

These considerations lead, in addition, to what might be called a psychic/emotional curriculum. In assessing what is most important for a child to learn in the process of educational growth, we consider certain psychic conditions that we need to help the child attain. The objectives of this curriculum are usually pursued simultaneously with those of the more traditional curriculum. Their attainment is often essential to the satisfactory completion of the traditional curriculum and at times, is even a precondition for it.

Erikson's conceptualization has been useful in organizing an understanding of what typical objectives of such a psychic curriculum might be.[1] Within the framework of the "average expectable environment," he postulates eight stages of life, during each of which there is a critical task that the growing individual has to master before proceeding successfully to the next stage. These tasks involve the integration of the demands of the inner world with those of the external world. How this integration at each stage is achieved is a basic factor in our ability to master later developmental tasks and in the formation of our character.

At each of these eight stages of development the inner world of the biological and emotional psyche is different, and is developing as outlined by Freud in his theory of the stages of psychosexual development. For example, the month-old is primarily moved by oral needs, the year-old by anal needs, and the adolescent by sexual needs. At the same time, Erikson suggests, there is a social timetable; the expectations of the growing self's environment also change. What the family and community provide and expect of an individual is different at every age. In these changing social expectations there are similar issues in all human development in all human environments. That is, every human being confronts an environment with similar expectations for particular ages. Every infant of the world is transported and fed; every adolescent of the world is expected to perform some task. This environment Erikson calls the "average expectable environment," and he describes its basic components at each of the eight stages that he postulates. According to this theory, the problems that the individual and society have to contend with are universal, but there is variation among societies as to how they are solved. The environment is presented by those closest to the child, but the nature of even the intimate environment of mother and child is influenced by the society and culture in which they live.

The way in which the individual masters the task of a given stage determines the ability to go on to the tasks of the next stage. It makes a significant contribution to a sense of self and becomes a more or less lasting part of character. Erikson suggests that the infant who does not learn to be trusting is very likely to become an overly suspicious adult; the latency child who does not succeed in learning becomes a person with feelings of inferiority.

The tasks about which he writes are ego tasks, and their mastery is an ego mastery. Our students who suffer from ego deficiencies have not been able to master these tasks. Whether the cause is an inborn deficit or a deficit acquired because the demands of the external world have been insurmountable has not been the subject of our explorations. Erikson's formulations are useful to us both in understanding the problems of our children and in developing methods of overcoming them.

From the perspective of his theory, our students have come to us because they have not been able to contend with the demands of the average expectable environment. A major part of our treatment is, therefore, to present them with a very different average expectable environment that they can master. As they do so we change the expectations, just as in the natural process of growth the expectations of the environment change, and the growing person, having mastered a given stage, moves on to new challenges and experiences.

All of our students have been unable to adapt. According to our understanding of the psychoanalytic view, the ego is the psychic agent of adaptation. When there is a problem in adaptation our approach is to concentrate not on the adaptation but on the ability to adapt, which is governed by the ego. So our efforts are concentrated on strengthening the ego. If we create an environment the expectations of which a student is able to meet, the ego will grow and become strengthened, and it will continue to grow as we change the expectations in line with the individual's developmental capabilities and provide the learning and support needed in order to meet the changing expectations.

Erikson's theory is valuable in helping us to identify at what stage the ability of a child's ego to adapt, to meet the demands of the environment, was overstressed. All of psychoanalytic theory helps us to understand what demands from inner forces were impinging on the ego. With this understanding we can act in such a way as to reduce excessive demands from both the inner and the outer worlds. The ego is then confronted with a job that is manageable and, therefore, can become strong and grow in doing its job. In everyday terms, our children have all been failures in life; in an environment that they can master, and in which they can feel successful, they are able to develop confidence and self-esteem and to grow.

Erikson's theory is also valuable in helping us to understand the components of the average expectable environment, to understand what the necessary tasks of human life are that a person has to master in order to live successfully. While at first we present an environment that is at the mastery level of our disturbed young people, this environment has to change gradually so that the ego gets appropriate exercise on the road to mastery of the ever-changing tasks of life. In the Orthogenic School we can control a whole environment. In more ordinary, less controlled environments, the same principle is valuable for those who help guide the development of others. That is, we always need to look both at the inner demands of an individual's biological and psychic needs and at the external demands of the environment, assess the individual's ability to cope with them, and do what we can to modify demands and develop the individual's capacity to cope.

I will now go through the first five stages of Erikson's scheme—that will bring us through adolescence—and give some examples of how we use his model to understand some of our students' difficulties and to provide a therapeutic learning environment—that is, how we find manageable jobs for the ego.

The first issue that every human being must resolve, according to the theory, is that of basic trust. This issue, of course, is not addressed by the infant on an intellectual level, but on a nonverbal, primitive, and very pervasive level. It is often reflected in physiological ways. It is not only *that* needs are met, but *how* they are met that determines the degree of trust an infant can have. Since during that period the major mode of experiencing and the area of investment of libidinal energy is oral, in the environment that we create at the School to rework the experience of trust, we concentrate a great deal on food and nurturing. As we do this, we take into account that the basic trust is not only trust in the environment that it will provide the needs of the child, but trust in the child's own ability to meet these needs.

At the School there is always food available that the child is able to get without the help of another person. In this way the anxiety of possibly not being fed never has to be suffered. It may seem strange that children in the rich land of the United States have this anxiety. But the anxiety does not have to do with the abundance of food, it has to do with the reliability of access to it. An infant may be provided with the best of milk and other infant foods, but if they are provided inconsistently, then anxiety about being fed can be engendered. There are debates as to which method of nursing is best: demand feeding, in which the infant is nursed when it asks by crying; or scheduled feeding, in which the infant is nursed at scheduled hours. As long as either is done fairly consistently so that the infant is fed reliably, trust can develop. Access has to do with more than timing. A mother who is tense or distracted may be unobservant or otherwise not in tune with the infant, so that the feeding may go badly. When one talks with mothers and observes infants, one finds that infants are very different from each other. Some are naturally vigorous suckers, others need to have their sucking reflexes stimulated. An anxious new mother may believe that a cranky infant is rejecting her or not know how to stimulate a passive baby, and the nursing experience can then be very frustrating.

We believe that children do not have to have elaborate food or large quantities of food, but they do have to feel that they can easily satisfy their hunger. If a child has to ask an adult for food, when that child has felt the caretaker to be out of tune with these needs, that child might well feel as though deprived of food. The quality of experience surrounding the food is of great importance in establishing the sense of trust. In our setting, the staff member who lovingly sprinkled sugar on plain bread for each of her students was much more effective in developing a relationship of trust than the one who brought soft drinks and expensive meats and left them on the table to be taken by whoever wanted them. It is very important to work out between staff member and child how that child will be able to *feel* well-fed, as well as nutritionally to *be* well-fed.

Though this issue is ordinarily worked out and a balance established in the first months of life, it is possible, and in the case of our youngsters, necessary, for a reworking to take place later in life. Frequently the balance established for these young people has been heavily on the side of mistrust, a balance and attitude which usually prevents them from successfully proceeding through the next stages of development. A thirteen-year-old adolescent came to us with a diagnosis of character disorder. She and her parents were extremely antagonistic. She had accused them of child abuse, and they in turn told us many stories of her delinquency and lack of concern for anyone else. On her first visit with us she commented on our generosity in serving her cheese and crackers. In her first year she could be satisfied in the evening only when her counselor would make a sandwich specially for her. Throughout this time she would complain to us of the stinginess of her parents in withholding food and giving only very "cheap" presents. She talked in this way even though her mother would often send food that she had baked specially for the girl. After a long time of seeing us as good feeders and her parents as bad she finally began to develop trust and could begin to see and believe that her parents actually had tried to feed her, but that she had been unable to perceive it, because their particular way of doing it was not in tune with her way of receiving.

It is of great importance that the teacher be part of the process of establishing trust. Our students are often not able to take anything in from their teachers until trust is established. The principle of availability of food extends to the classroom, and the practice of students eating lunch with their teacher contributes to the development of a relationship of trust. Evidence for the interrelationship of food and trust is at times subtle, but at times is quite striking. An anorexic girl would become upset and eat less if her teacher did not attend strongly enough to what she was eating, and at times would run screaming from the dining room in reaction to what she perceived to be inattentiveness. This girl was not able to even begin to learn in class until her teacher had, literally, held her by the hand for months to be sure to keep her safe.

In addition to providing such nurturing experiences, responsive to the particular needs of the individual, the environment must be accepting of the need for this kind of nurturing. In society at large, an adolescent would be ridiculed for accepting the kind of care that many of our adolescents need in order to develop trust that they can get their primitive needs met. And in society at large the caregiver would be criticized as infantilizing that adolescent. We try to make it clear that ours is a specialized environment in that respect, and that it need not be a blow to the young person's self-esteem to be babied. In society at large, the expectable environment for an infant is one that responds favorably to an infant who drinks from a bottle, and whose mother ties its shoes; for an adolescent, it is one that responds with criticism to a teenager who drinks from a baby bottle or whose shoes are tied by another. For some of our teenagers, being able to get such care without criticism from their environment and without giving up higher-level functioning has been essential to their emotional growth. Though in our classrooms the highest level of functioning is expected, this expectation is to the best of our knowledge and ability assessed in terms of the child's developmental level.

The next stage that Erikson talks about is that of autonomy versus shame and doubt. This stage usually occurs at the time of what Freud referred to as the anal stage. At this time not only is the libidinal energy focused around the anus but, at least as important, the child's physiological development has progressed to the point of muscular control, including control of the sphincter muscles. The environment at this age is one that expects some self-control on the part of the young child in many areas, including that of urinary and bowel control. It is, therefore, typically the age of toilet training. How this is done, what accomodation is worked out between parent and child, has a significant influence on personality development. Developing the feeling of being in control of body functions in this stage will give the child basically the feeling of being an autonomous person. If, however, in conflict with parents who try to impose too harshly their control, the child is unable to develop bodily control, feelings of shame will develop. At this stage the child needs the appropriate doses of imposed control and guidance. If the environment does not impose enough control and support, the child is likely to fail, having neither judgement nor power to exert self-control. Unless taught not to, a toddler may walk into a dangerous street and get hurt. Having such an experience—that self-selected and self-effected action may lead to hurt—can engender feelings of shame and doubt.

Children that we see who have had unsuccessful experiences at this stage are often those who most loudly assert how much in control they are. They are often those who show most uncontrolled physical behavior by an almost constant need for movement. Fairly often they are enuretic. In the structuring of our environment we address the issue first by having the environment very clear and manageable, including, as has been described, outlines of the day that are unchanging so that students know what will be happening at what time each day. Life at the School is predictable. Within this predictable environment we try to give our students as much experience as possible in making good choices. For example, each student is allowed to choose a birthday activity. The choice, however, is among activities that can be successful. If the student has no ideas, we suggest alternatives which we know will be manageable and enjoyable, so that the student will have the feeling and experience of success when in control.

One of our boys for whom the issue of autonomy was of critical importance was able to be significantly helped in learning by our attention to this issue. This boy's feelings of autonomy had been severely handicapped by a very early bone fracture that had imposed pain and limitations on his motility. In addition, an explosive, alcoholic father had imposed either overly harsh or overly lenient controls. Though he was a very bright boy, for a long time he would not learn what anyone else presented to him. When he himself selected a topic and had a teacher's undivided attention, he could learn. After many months of acceding to this mode of learning, his teacher was able to interest him in a topic that the teacher had selected but that was very obviously related to the boy's interest. Since he had developed the feeling that he could be in control of his learning, he was able to permit his teacher also to have some control. Thus he was finally able to believe that letting another have joint control did not mean entirely forfeiting his control.

The third stage in Erikson's scheme is that of initiative versus guilt. This stage is coincident with the phallic stage of psychosexual development. Though what I have to say about our application of theory at this stage does not distinguish between boys and girls, I think it is important to note that it is generally agreed that the traditional theory of psychosexual development, including the designation of this level as phallic, does not adequately deal with the development of girls. That libidinal energy is focused around the genital area is supported by observations of four-year-olds. However, it is not focused only on the male genitals, as the name implies.

At this stage the child is more aggressively assertive. The environment expects motility in the world and at the same time presents limitations. In this interactive process, guilt is a significant component. The balance of healthy initiative and healthy guilt is important for the development of an individual who can freely and actively pursue goals without infringing on the rights of others. If the environment is overly critical of the assertiveness of the child, crippling guilt can develop. On the other hand, without some kind of check from the environment a person can grow without respect for the needs and desires of anyone else.

An aspect of our program that directly addresses the problems of this stage of development is physical education. Though our children are physically without handicaps, they frequently are impeded from using their bodies because of overwhelming anxiety about the integrity of their bodies and because of overwhelming fear of what they might do if they exercise their initiative physically. Being able to successfully use their bodies and to physically play without doing harm to themselves or anyone else is a most deeply effective demonstration both of the integrity of their bodies and of the possibility of safely exerting initiative. Because of the intensity of the anxieties about injury, we are very careful to modify our activities to reduce the likelihood of physical harm. When any injury takes place, we take it very seriously and explore the reasons for its having happened. We also are very careful to reduce the competitive aspects of play to manageable proportions and to modify our games so that fear of being beaten and fear of hurting others are not inhibiting. In this way, the playing of games is a good opportunity for our students to learn how to be vigorously aggressive without hurting other people.

The critical issue in the fourth stage of development, according to Erikson, is that of industry versus inferiority. This stage coincides with the time of latency. In all cultures children at this age are expected to begin to acquire the tools of society. In our society, children do not enter the world of work, but the world of school, which eventually leads to mastery of the world of work. It is at this stage that the average expectable environment very clearly goes beyond the family and consists of some of the institutions of society. Erikson suggests that

A PLACE TO LEARN

whether the child is able to master the tasks presented by the world of work, in our society by the world of school, determines the view of self as a capable person. The child who is not able to learn in school is likely to suffer in general from feelings of inferiority.

The school class is therefore a very important component in the environment that we create at the Orthogenic School. In terms of Erikson's framework it is essential that it be separate and distinct and that it present a clear learning task. We make use of our knowledge of the students' capabilities, interests, and desires to provide tasks that they will attend to and master. Because of the importance to a sense of self and sense of competence, class attendance from 9:00 A.M. to 3:00 P.M. daily is expected, even when a student is not ready to engage in academic learning.

The crucial problem to be resolved at the next stage is that of identity versus role diffusion. This stage comes at the time of adolescence. At this age, coinciding with the beginning surge of adult sexuality, the young person is trying to find a sense of self apart from family. Society has the expectation that adolescents begin to decide on their work roles. This task has to be mastered by a growing person in any society, but in some societies it is more difficult than in others. In our society two major difficulties are, first, the long period of training before the adolescent has real adult responsibilities and, second, the great range of career choices available for the majority of adolescents.

Though our students have not mastered the conflicts of the four previous stages, they are still subject to both the inner and outer pressures of this stage. They want to define themselves apart from their families. One of the ways that young people typically attempt to do this is by joining a peer group and testing their ideas in that society. Peer groups can be healthy and valuable for this kind of testing, but can be dangerous if used as a vehicle for testing harmful practices or as an alliance against society. With our knowledge of the importance of testing, we try to provide classes and activities that will address the issues that are important to adolescents. For example, we have had a class in social anthropology for a group of adolescents to study other cultures, both animal and human, and to discuss some of their social practices. They become fascinated with the mating practices of animals and draw analogies to their own mating practices. They can discuss and see the value of traditional rituals in more primitive societies—for example, the ordeals that young men must go through in some societies in order to enter adult manhood—and can understand that such rituals deal with problems with which they themselves contend. Though our students through most of their residence with us are too afraid to think of a professional role, in this kind of discussion they can consider with their friends their roles as members of society.

I have so far outlined some aspects of what might be considered a psychic curriculum. The theory of psychoanalytic ego psychology can also contribute to the development of an academic curriculum and to the selection of its subject matter. This topic will be amplified in a later chapter.

We can derive from psychoanalytic theory, as well as from common sense, that in order to learn, a person has to pay attention. There are many things that make a person likely to pay attention. A strong desire to achieve something (if one wants to be a great scientist, one must pay attention to studying chemistry), a desire to win approval (if one thinks one's parents value learning, one pays attention to work in school to gain more love), and fear (if one will get beaten for not learning the times tables, one might pay attention to them) may all provide reasons for attentiveness to a particular subject. A somewhat different kind of reason can be that the subject itself attracts that attention. In psychoanalytic terms this means that the subject is highly cathected: if one is presented with material that has psychic energy connected to it, one will easily pay attention and learn. That we pay attention to those things that are most highly cathected was demonstrated to me most effectively in one of my early psychology classes, when a professor pointed out how easily we can find our own names on a list. I have often had the experience of watching an official pore over a long list of names very carefully trying to find my name, which to him is hidden in a confusion of similar letters; I can see it in an instant, as though it were lit up in neon lights.

At one time in my career I worked for a man in charge of a project to develop learning material for preschool culturally deprived children. These were children from low-income families which had not taught them to develop the perceptual skills necessary to be successful in school learning. The government had given the group money to develop material for teaching these children, before they entered regular public school, the kinds of skills that middle class children in the United States usually develop at home. The reasoning was that the lack of the skills was a primary cause of failure in school. This project was part of the Head Start movement, which was based on findings regarding the importance of early learning. It of course was very much in keeping with Erikson's conceptualization of the timing of entry into the world of society and work and the importance of acquiring its tools. The principles that were being employed in this project were the principles of learning theory. The children were shown stimuli at intervals that would help them to learn and were given reinforcement at the appropriate times. The principal investigator for the project hired me to join the work because he thought my orientation, very different from his, could help in the problem they were having. The problem was that the children were not looking at the material: all the valid reinforcement schedules and the other means employed in keeping with behavioral theory were not effective, since the children were not paying attention. He wanted me to help develop subject material that would interest the children (in my terms, material that would be highly cathected for the children).

Some years earlier than this, Sylvia Ashton-Warner, in a most imaginative way and without benefit of any psychological theory, came to similar conclusions in her work with native children in New Zealand.[2] The children with whom she worked were also of beginning school age and were also not from the learned part of society. They could not learn at all from the regular school books. She therefore introduced them to learning by creating individual textbooks for them. She would start out with each child by finding for that child what she called the key word. This was a "one look" word, a word that the child would remember after having had just one look at it. She would make a word card for that word, and the child would remember it the next day, and the next, and forever after. These were not the conventional words of a beginning reading book. They most frequently came from the emotional life of the child, and could include words of violence and anger as well as words of love and joy. They were evidently words that were highly cathected. From each child's words she could then develop the individual text for the child.

We have found that at the beginning of learning it is especially important to find for the child material that is highly cathected. When this material is mastered, it is then possible for the learning itself to become cathected, and the child can go on to master other kinds of learning that are not in themselves cathected. We have frequently had this experience when we have sent students out to study in colleges or other educational institutions outside of the school. If the student is generally unsure, we always advise taking a course that may not be required, but is closely related to the student's interest. The student therefore easily attends to the material and can more easily master it. The experience of taking a course becomes positively charged and facilitates success in other courses that the student subsequently takes.

Creating material for an individual student that is based on intimate knowledge of the student is one way of applying the principle and insuring attention. Another way is working with the student to select material that is appropriately cathected. A boy who could not pay attention to reading books could pay attention to signs, because not being able to read signs and labels had gotten him into trouble. He had once taken an overdose of aspirin, not being able to read the warning label on the bottle. By asking the meaning of signs on the street and labels on boxes, bottles, and cans he acquired enough of a sight-reading vocabulary to be able to read relatively simple books. The experience of reading then brought him enough pleasure to be able to pay attention to it, and he became a voracious reader.

We have also been able to use our knowledge of the psyche to choose material that would have value for a whole class. For example, we know that many children are fascinated by weather. We believe that this is so because of certain characteristics of weather. Weather seems to express affect—a thunderstorm seems angry, as though giants on high are shouting and fighting, and a sunny day seems friendly, as though warm emotionally as well as physically. Weather is also unpredictable. The fascination, we can speculate, is that if one could only predict the storms and sunshine of those giants on high who make the climate of our physical surroundings, one might be able to predict the storms and sunshine of those giants on earth, one's parents, who make the climate of our emotional surroundings. With these issues in mind we have had successful units on the weather. One teacher taught about weather to a class of five very disturbed children, including one autistic boy. All of these children had great trouble learning, but all learned how to make some basic kinds of weather predictions. The autistic boy began to learn to read; his first text consisted of the scientific names of the different types of clouds.

As well as the nature of content that can facilitate learning, it is possible also to derive from psychoanalytic theory the nature of content that will be likely to produce impediments to learning. Material that arouses intense anxiety is likely to interfere with learning. Particularly at the beginning of learning, we try to avoid material that will make the student excessively anxious. We find, for example, that children who have suffered loss, perhaps through parental divorce or another kind of separation, while having no trouble in mathematics with addition and multiplication, may have particular difficulty with subtraction and division. So we try to arrange the order of their studies to avoid subtraction and division as long as possible, until their security about loss has been strengthened through other means.

Biology is a subject matter that contains very highly cathected material—what could be more cathected than one's own body? Biology also contains much material that produces very great anxiety. Anything about sickness, for example, has to be modified to build in enough reassurance so that the students' anxiety does not prevent them from learning. A most striking example occurred when the teacher of a small class of disturbed adolescents, who were working very well together, began a unit on genetics. The teacher had not adequately assessed the impact that this unit would have on her students and presented it to them as she had all other units. Because of their intense anxiety about the possible hereditary nature of their own emotional disturbances, the adolescents were unable to manage the material, and a usually well-behaved and interested class dissolved into chaos.

At the Orthogenic School the curriculum for each child and each classroom is decided upon individually. Each class usually studies one to three subjects as à group. The group gains a feeling of coherence and has the experience of learning together. Since the groups are heterogenous, the topics for group study have to be selected from those that can be approached at various levels. There are a variety of subjects that are amenable to this kind of treatment. The teacher usually presents a core lesson appropriate for all students and then assigns individual lessons at the learning level of each student. We have, for example, had a successful geography unit done in this way, in which a less competent child colored in pictures of a particular country, while a more sophisticated child drew a complicated map.

In planning the curriculum we consider the same basic issues as most educational planners: the child's age and current level of knowledge and cognitive development. We also must consider the normative curriculum of the area the child is likely to enter when ready to master the world outside of the Orthogenic School. However, before we can begin to present this kind of curriculum, we have to understand what the psychic curriculum of each child should be—what emotional learning first has to take place. That psychic curriculum has to continue to be a part of our planning as long as a student is at the School. We want to be sure that our students know, when they leave the School, what other young people know. But more important, we want them to understand that learning and knowledge are of value to them in achieving what they want to achieve. If they understand the latter, they will more easily acquire the former. Particularly at the beginning of learning, we utilize what we know of the child's psychology, both on the basis of general developmental level and on the basis of particular psychic needs, to select subject matter that will be highly cathected and will therefore facilitate learning. Such highly cathected subject matter, being emotionally very relevant to the student, gives the student the feeling that learning is of personal value. Throughout the learning experience, even through those times that the student is committed to learning, we try to select subject matter that will in some way be helpful to the student in the mastery of critical psychological issues (like the unit for adolescents on primitive tribes).

In summary, with care first to their mastery of psychological learning and to their protection from undue anxiety evoked by learning, children can be attracted to learning because of its significance to them and can then utilize it to solve not only cognitive but also emotional dilemmas.

FIVE

The Art of Being an Understanding Teacher

The teachers of the Orthogenic School are, of course, the ones who struggle to answer for each of their students the questions raised at the beginning of the preceding chapter: what are the emotional preconditions of learning, what are the emotional facilitators of learning, what are the emotional impediments to learning, and what kind of learning can contribute to the emotional well-being of the child. At the same time, of course, they must organize and present the actual learning tasks. In this chapter I will address some issues that are critical in the ability to arrive at the answers, or at least at closer and closer approximations of the answers, to those questions.

At any given time there have been five to seven teachers at the Orthogenic School. They have to work together, and they usually manage to do so. They are dependent on each other to help with difficult children or situations, to share facilities, to plan recesses, to take each other's students during vacation periods, and, we hope, to be mutually supportive. During the period under discussion they have ranged in age from twenty-two to fifty, in educational level from bachelor's degree to doctorate, in teacher training from Montessori to cognitive psychology to none, in experience from intensive work with severely disturbed youngsters to regular classroom teaching to none, in size from tall and skinny to short and fat, in countenance from plain to ravishing, and in activity level from athletically vigorous to sedentary. I can find in these dimensions no way to characterize the typical teacher at the School.

For quite a few years all of our teacher applicants came to us either by their own initiative (many had become interested through Bettelheim's publications) or through a suggestion of a colleague or friend. Though we advertised to every college in the country for counselors, it did not occur to me to advertise for teachers when we had openings. When someone came on the basis of the School's reputation, it was usually important to discover what the person's expectation was. A commonly held, erroneous belief that would mean disaster for a teacher, if left uncorrected, was that the teacher was to be a therapist. An untrained person who wanted to learn to teach was always a much better risk than a trained teacher who wanted to learn therapy. Though our students need understanding, they need it in the context of structure and learning.

Through this unsystematic process we obtained some excellent teachers. In fact, the quality in general was so high that when the state began to insist that we have a certain percentage of teachers with credentials, I worried that we wouldn't be able to maintain our quality. However, we found that while having appropriate credentials is no insurance that a person has the other appropriate qualities, neither does it prevent a person from having them. And of course, it represents additional useful training and skill.

I have sometimes pondered this issue—the reason for the great success of the untrained teacher. We have had a number of wonderful teachers who were first counselors and then, without any formal training, became teachers. Two former students of the School became teachers, one with formal training and one without. It has always seemed to me that the intense investment of the staff members in their own learning and growth is a very powerful curative factor, to the extent that they serve as objects of identification to their charges. I believe that this factor cannot be overestimated in assessing the value of the counselors to the students: the counselors are by self-definition engaged in an intensive learning process. I ponder whether there might not be a loss in this respect when staff members' need to learn is less intense, as might be the case with teachers who are both experienced in teaching and have substantial understanding of disturbed children. Of course, it is likely that anyone who elects to work at a school that is part of a university and thus, almost by definition, is devoted to all levels of learning, does so in part because of interest in learning. Therefore, though the teacher's intensity of commitment might be somewhat diminished, it is still a significant force. The benefit for the students of having a more highly skilled, experienced, and knowledgeable teacher, as opposed to having the motivating force of a highly invested role model, would be difficult to measure. Perhaps as a result of this orientation toward learning and growing, our good teachers have stayed at the School during this period only from three to six years.

Teachers at the School work longer hours than most teachers (since they eat with their classes and usually have recess and physical education with them), their days off are fewer (since class is in session on all but the most important holidays and through December and the summer), and their pay is less than public school pay. I asked one of our teachers why a good teacher would want such a job. He replied that it was in part because he enjoyed the freedom to teach as he saw fit, which he might not have had in a public school (but which he actually had also had in his former position). What he described as being the truly distinctive value was that which in a way was also so burdensome—the totality of the responsibility for the growth of his students, not just for their academic achievements. This responsibility, while more of a burden than the usual tasks assigned to teachers, allows more opportunity to make a significant difference in the lives of these children. The teacher has the responsibility for a relationship with each student and for all aspects of the student's life while in the classroom. If the child is in distress, the teacher does not hand the problem over to a therapist, but struggles to help the child manage the distress in the context of the classroom. While from the teacher's point of view it would be easier in the short run to hand the child over to someone else, it is likely to be far more gratifying to work the situation through with the child.

The foregoing description is an attempt at a general understanding of the ingredients necessary, from our point of view, to make a good teacher. They are ingredients that, though I believe they can be taught, I've never made any attempt to teach to our staff; I have consciously or unconsciously expected or hoped that they would be present. My discussion now turns to two other components, which I have tried to teach, in various settings: first, the issue of understanding, and second, the selection of curriculum.

All teachers, whether in a residential institution for disturbed youngsters or in a regular classroom, deal with psychological issues, whether they like it or not and whether they know it or not. Children do not leave their psyches at home when they come to class. Even those in treatment refuse to leave their psyches in their therapists' offices. Nor do teachers leave their psyches at home. For example, on the first school day in January, teachers have to deal with the effects of a one- or two-week vacation from school, the disappointments or elations of Christmas, the letdown from the excitement of the holidays, and the anxiety of what the new semester will hold. They have to deal with these issues because, no matter what the subject matter, the children have them inside. Ignoring them is as much a way of dealing with them as talking about them for hours. The problem is to determine which of the ways, if either, is more likely to enhance the education of the children. Talking about such matters may not seem to be in line with most educational goals, but if they are absorbing a child, they might prevent the learning of anything else. When a teacher is able to find a way of dealing with psychological issues appropriately, the children feel comfortable and learn. When asked what he liked so much about a favorite and very effective teacher, one little boy said that it was that he understood kids so well. This little boy worked harder for his teacher than he ever had before in school. He was delighted when he was given a higher level spelling book; when offered this honor the previous year, he had said, "What do I want that for? I have enough trouble with the book I have now." Since his teacher understood him, he felt that what the teacher valued must have some merit, and so he valued it also. Thus he both felt comfortable and learned. In other words, a good teacher has to be understanding: not an understanding *person*, but an understanding *teacher*. Explicitly or implicitly the good teacher knows that the child needs both understanding and a clear structure to be secure and to grow.

In my experience as instructor and consultant to teachers in a variety of settings that included a range of intensity and supervision, psychoanalytic ego psychology has proved to be a useful framework for helping to develop both the understanding and the teaching of the child, psyche and all. Of the three settings from which examples will be drawn, the most intensive was a series of meetings with teachers at the

Orthogenic School. The least intensive was a six-week graduate course entitled "Psychological Problems in the Classroom," meeting for two-hour periods twice a week that I
taught every summer for several years at the University of
Chicago. A middle level of intensity was a number of seminars each week with groups of nursery school teachers-in-
training, at the junior college affiliated with a psychoanalytically oriented nursery school and day care center in
Los Angeles.

The meetings with the teachers at the Orthogenic School
were small: there were only six or seven teachers. The meetings were once a week (the teachers also attended several
other meetings every week with the rest of the staff) and were
primarily for the purpose of developing psychologically sound
curricula.

The student teachers at the nursery school and day care
center were involved in a two-year course that combined a
daily practicum at the nursery school with course work. As
part of the course they were obliged to attend a weekly seminar to discuss problems of student teaching. In the practicum
each student worked with one head teacher for a semester and
then changed, so as to have experience with all preschool ages.
There were about twenty children in a class. The students had
opportunity to know the children they worked with fairly
well. The seminars were small, and the students involved saw
each other daily.

The graduate course ranged in size from fifteen to thirty-
five students over the years. The students taught in a wide
variety of settings, from nursery school to college English
classes, and had a wide variety of experience, since they
ranged from student teacher to retired teacher.

In the meetings with each of the groups, the central question addressed was how to be an understanding teacher. In
one such meeting with student teachers, a problem was presented by a young lady who thought she was understanding,
wanted to be a teacher, but was stymied by a little girl's persistent, teasing habit of running down the hall calling her
"fatso." As one of the counselors at the Orthogenic School
put it so well, "It's easy enough to be understanding when a
kid is lying on his bed crying about how bad he feels. It's a lot

harder when he's attacking you." The student teacher's problem demonstrates that, before considering how to understand psychological issues and what, as a teacher, to do with that understanding, it is necessary to discuss some things that stand in the way of understanding, those things that prevent us from doing even what we know exactly how to do. For example, to understand another one has to think of the other's point of view. But this student teacher could not possibly begin to think of the point of view of the child who was calling her "fatso." She was too hurt and angry, and so she simply wanted to stop the child. I gave her no advice on how to do so, but instead asked her why she was so hurt by the child's calling her "fatso." The student teacher (and the rest of the class) thought that this was a ridiculous question—of course, anyone's feelings would have been hurt. I pointed out that if there was nothing wrong with being fat, and I saw nothing wrong with being fat, then there was nothing to be hurt about in being called "fatso." The student teacher, who *was* fat, did not maintain that there was anything wrong with being fat, but did maintain that being hurt was a perfectly reasonable reaction, and, in fact, the only possible reaction. Furthermore, she thought that I was being rather cruel to imply that her reaction was unreasonable. There the discussion ended. By the next class period, the student teacher's attitude toward me had changed. (She subsequently became very devoted to me.) The problem of name calling had vanished. We can speculate that when the student teacher no longer experienced being called "fatso" as an attack, the child immediately could tell. Since the child no longer received an angry response she had less motivation to tease, and she could go on to express herself in other ways.

What had been done was to question the assumption that the teacher's reaction to the action of the child was the only possible reaction. Contrary to the belief of the student and her classmates, everyone would not be hurt by being called "fatso." A thin person would not be, nor would someone who liked being fat, who was called that by someone who also liked it. The student teacher was, of course, hurt because of her own negative feelings about being fat. At times it is helpful for a teacher to explore such inner feelings. However, that would not have been appropriate for such a seminar, nor was it necessary for this teacher. My stance was based on the psychoanalytic assumption that whatever a person does serves that person usefully; when one is fat, one gains something very valuable from it, and so cannot feel only bad about it. Thus, insistence that there was no reason to feel bad about being called "fatso," was supporting the positive in the student's desire to be fat. I believe that it was because of the implicit recognition of this that the student teacher was able to handle the name calling (and that she became so devoted to me).

While it is often difficult for us to recognize the possibility of change in our own reactions when they are questioned, it is often possible to learn from another's situation. At the Orthogenic School one staff member was stymied by his reaction to an adolescent boy telling him that he was "worth less than nothing" to the boy. The staff member could see no other reaction than to be angry at the boy's terrible arrogance. He could think of no situation when he himself would say such a thing. Another staff member could, however, imagine that she might have said such a thing, in a situation where she had felt terribly hurt and disappointed by someone she cared for very much and felt powerless to influence. At the time of her response to the other staff member, the issue had no immediate pertinence to her. However, not long after, a boy called her "nigger"; she was suddenly able to stop feeling put down and hurt by it, and to realize that he was insulting her out of his own feeling of being defeated. She was then able to tell him that neither of them was going to be defeated, that she would teach him how to master the problem (building with Lego blocks) that seemed to be defeating him.

Though a neutral reaction might not lead one to know what to do about an issue such as name calling, at least it is unlikely to make it worse. One can then make use of suggestions from other people. A very disturbed boy was calling two staff members, a man and a woman, "bloody vagina." The younger staff member, the woman, felt criticized and hurt by the name; the more experienced staff member, the man, was curious. When the boy called such names he seemed to be evoking a vivid image in his own mind. Since it was a disembodied image, it was suggested that the staff member ask, "To whom, then, do

I belong?" Both staff members could intellectually understand the value in doing so: by asking the question, we were following the fantasy with a question that would encourage elaboration and, therefore, understanding. However, only the man could effectively ask the question, because the woman still felt hurt. The boy replied to the question that the counselor belonged "to Jacqui" (the Director), and he proceeded to complain vigorously about me. He never called the male staff member "vagina" again. We might speculate that "bloody vagina" referred to menstruation, a subject about which an eleven-year-old boy might be both very curious and very anxious, but which carries a strong taboo in our society. We might also speculate that a man, with some experience and, therefore, freedom from the taboo, might have empathy with a boy's curiosity about it. The boy's reaction indicated that there were important feelings behind what he said, which the staff member's encouragement permitted him to express. On the other hand, he continued to say such things to the woman staff member for a much longer time, as she could only gradually stop feeling attacked. We again might speculate that dealing with this social taboo is a much more difficult issue for a woman.

In all the instances described, the teacher's problem was one of feeling attacked and hurt by a child's verbal aggressions. When the teacher could be helped to experience the name calling as something other than an attack, it ceased to be a problem. Help was given in one case by providing support for the teacher's view of herself—that being fat is not bad. In the second case, the opportunity was provided for the staff member to learn, through considering her own experience, that putting down someone else is an expression of one's own insecurities. Once the view of name calling as an attack had been challenged and changed, it was even possible for the teacher to make use of the name calling to be helpful: in one instance, in a learning situation of mastering an external task; in another instance, in a therapeutic situation of mastering an internal task.

This discussion should not be interpreted to mean that we are never critical of a youngster's verbal aggression. From both the student's and the teacher's points of view, it is important

that the student develop control of aggressive, negative behavior. When, however, we have very strong emotional reactions, we frequently are not able to exert control in a consistent, forthright manner.

In order to be an understanding teacher, one has to be able
to see things from the student's point of view. But in the day-
to-day life of the classroom many things interfere with the
ability to do this. It was, therefore, pressing in all three kinds of
meetings to help teachers with those anxieties and feelings
that stood in the way of their gaining or utilizing this understanding. It is never easy to admit to being hurt by a child,
being angry at a child, feeling inadequate in relationship to a
child; but it is certainly easier to do so in a small, ongoing
seminar than in a large, short-term class. It was usually not
possible to do much more in the class than to let the teacher
who was perturbed by feelings of anger at a child know that
experiencing such anger was by no means a unique experience. While this assurance at least offers some relief from guilt,
a teacher needs to be able to gain more perspective on such
reactions in order to be able to be free enough of the anger or
anxiety to do something positive. There are areas of interference with understanding that could be dealt with even in
the less-supportive situation of the large class meeting. Many
times a teacher is blinded by ordinary routines and expectations. A teacher of younger children was concerned about the
rowdiness of the boys when it came time to put away the
blocks. She complained about how difficult it was to get them
to do so, and how much trouble they got into in the process.
When asked why they had to put the blocks away at that
particular time, she said that there was no reason other than
that of the established routine. She then realized that she could
be more flexible about the ending of block time, to allow for a
closure of whatever project the boys were working on. The
teacher experienced this as a remarkable insight that was extremely valuable to her in her work. It seems that the value was
in questioning an assumption. Until asked why the block
building had to end at an arbitrary time, the teacher assumed
that it was necessary. Simply questioning this assumption enabled her to see another possibility.

Another teacher had been able to free herself of an assumption enough to act in the best way for a child, but doubted the rightness of her action. She described how a little boy had come to her class as a problem. He was absolutely no problem to her, as long as she kept him by her side. However, she was uneasy about what she was doing and felt that there was something wrong with it, because of the expectation that a child of his age should sit at his desk. This assumption was based on the notion that by this age a certain structure is usually developed that enables a child to be self-sustaining. She was assured that if the structure has not yet been attained, then the only sensible thing to do was to provide the necessary external support. Thus, automatic assumptions will sometimes interfere with seeing a sensible way of acting. Challenging such assumptions by simply asking a teacher to consider why they exist—why Thursday, for example, is scheduled in a certain way—has helped the teacher to develop sounder practices and to solve some classroom problems.

The foregoing has been a discussion of some of the issues that *interfere* with teachers' understanding of their students. Some of the ways teachers can *gain* understanding of their students are, of course, their own teachers, courses, colleagues, and books. There is much of importance that is not written in books, and of that which is, we have to decide what we should believe. Long before Freud, great writers and philosophers began teaching that there is a way, available to us all, to begin to understand the mind of another, and that is through trying to understand our own mind. According to psychoanalytic theory, while each of our minds is unique, all have certain elements in common. So, to have some notion of the way another person feels, we have only to put ourselves in the position of the other and try to imagine how we would feel in just that position. This, of course, is only the beginning of understanding. In addition to an idea of how the person feels, we have to have some idea of what the person needs and what would help the person to cope with the feeling.

In order to accustom the members of the large class to this way of thinking, they were asked to tell about how they had felt in a particular situation as a child. When they were asked about their attitudes toward math, as might be expected, some remembered loving it and some remembered hating it. Both groups gave the same answer as to why they had felt the way they did: because in math there is always a clear-cut right answer. To those who had liked math, it had been reassuring that they could if they worked at it eventually find what was right and what was wrong. To those who had disliked it, it had been distressing that one had to find the right answer, not approximately, but exactly; that if one could not find it absolutely and clearly, one was wrong.

That such recognition of feeling is only a beginning became very evident in one discussion of ability grouping. Class members were asked how they had felt about being grouped by ability when they were in grade school. Most of the students had been in the highest ability group; though they had liked the recognition, they were not particularly positive toward the idea of ability grouping. The one student in the class who had been in the lowest ability group spoke at some length about how bad she had felt about being one of the "dummies" of the class. She felt that being in the lowest group had done nothing beneficial for her, had not helped her learn, and only made her feel worse about herself. However, she was the only student in the class who used ability grouping in her own classroom; none of the others would even consider doing so. In the discussion which ensued she could make no connection between her bad feelings and the feelings of the students in her own class. Though this teacher could easily remember how she had felt, she could not really put herself in the place of her students. One might speculate that she did not have enough mastery of the experience for it to be useful in the service of others. The reminder of it produced the kind of distress to which she could not respond rationally. It therefore led her to do much as we all do when we repeat with our own children exactly those experiences that we hated most when our parents imposed them on us. Her behavior toward her own class can be explained as an effort on her part to master the degrading experience. Using ability grouping accomplished this in two ways. First, despite her statements that being in the lowest group did her no good, deep down she had to believe that such suffering as she had experienced must have been for some purpose; thus, to be a good teacher she had to use the same method. Second, for her to be in charge of exactly the situation in which she had felt so inadequate was the ultimate demonstration that she had mastery of it.

When an experience is not so strongly related to an as-yet-unresolved issue, the attempt to put oneself in the student's place is usually helpful. In the setting of the Orthogenic School the members of the staff ask themselves and each other to think of a time when they might do the same as the students. For example, when we were considering what, if anything, to do about one girl's sizable weight gain, one staff member said that she thought we should help her to lose weight because the girl didn't like the way she looked. When asked to give the evidence she had that the girl felt that way, she said, "Well, when she gets dressed she often asks J and me how we think she looks." When asked under what conditions the staff member herself asked others how she looked, the staff member noted that she did so when she felt insecure and wanted reassurance. When she really thought she looked bad she did not ask; she asked only if there was some possibility in her own mind that she looked good. It became immediately apparent to the staff member that she had been wrong about the girl's view of herself. The girl did not simply think that she looked bad; though she probably was insecure, she most likely thought that in some way she looked good.

Thus, imagining will help clarify the understanding of a situation. Of course, we can never be absolutely certain that our speculations are correct. Even when our imaginings do not lead to a precise understanding of the student, they are helpful, in that the staff member is assuming the perspective of the student and is therefore immediately on the side of the student.

Another way to begin to understand others is by watching precisely what they are doing. There are many situations where difficulties could be avoided if this were done. For example, a major trouble spot in most nursery school classrooms is the boys' play in the block corner. The teacher is usually occupied with the more controlled, "constructive" table activity, rather than watching the less structured and, therefore, more potentially explosive block activity. Teachers often do not watch disruptive children until they are disrupting. In the seminars with teachers-in-training, when participants were asked to describe what had happened before a child started misbehaving, they would, more often than not, not be able to do so. Even when teachers described certain children as acting up "all day long," it usually turned out that these children would be attended to when they were acting up and paid little or no attention when they were not. (This is often because the adults are so relieved that a problem child is quiet that they just let the child be.)

A teacher who watches learns the cues of the child and thus can tell when the child needs support or diversion. After being persistently asked to describe what has happened, a teacher begins automatically to pay more attention, and the acting up is reduced. At the Orthogenic School, where such questions are repeated frequently, we concentrate on watching and understanding the inception of disruptive behavior. The teachers learn to be watchful and perceptive and, as a result, to stop the acting up before it starts.

Intellectual understanding of another human being is not too hard to come by, but real understanding, the kind that is useful for a teacher in action, confronted by a class full of children, by disruptive behavior, and by lessons to present, is the result of a long, persistent process. At the end of a typical day of teaching difficult youngsters, no one is likely to appreciate being asked to think over and describe exactly what happened, or to imagine being in the place of the students. We ask such questions as much as we can, and it helps.

In considering the issue of psychologically sound teaching, the first question to be asked is the same from a psychological point of view as from a curricular point of view: "What are you trying to achieve?" The importance of clarifying one's purpose is evident in the psychological literature as well as in the curriculum literature. Bateson has described the double-bind, a situation wherein the parent makes conflicting demands on the child, so that complying with one demand necessitates doing the opposite of the other.[1] A most simple example occurs when a mother tells her child to go to the teacher or play with other children, while holding the youngster on her lap, enveloped in her arms. The verbal message is, "I want you to go," while the physical message is, "I want you to stay." The child is thus in a double-bind: complying with the one message means defying the other. Bateson suggests that a child pervasively put in such situations can become schizophrenic. Though we are not suggesting that a teacher's conflicting messages are likely to be so devastating, if a teacher says one thing and means another it can easily lead to a chaotic classroom. Frequently teachers are not clear as to their major goals, and often their goals are at variance with what they are actually doing. Asking them what they are trying to achieve, frequently is helpful in clarifying a troublesome area, because they are then more likely to think through what they are doing in terms of what they are trying to achieve. For example, one nursery school teacher said that she wanted to teach a child to tell another child that he did not like it when the second child hit him. She had an overall goal of increasing reliance on verbal skills. But as she discussed it, she said, "But it really doesn't do any good, it won't stop A from hitting him." In other words, her goal was one that she did not believe in. Recognizing this conflict, she was able to reevaluate both her goal and her actions.

At the Orthogenic School we have discussed the issue of teaching by asking questions. This didactic technique is frequently used but has some undesirable consequences. When some teachers ask a question, it is because they really want to know the *students'* answers. However, since most students have been subjected to this technique for years, they are convinced that any question asked by a teacher is to see if the students know the *teacher's* answer. One of our teachers was having a difficult time in her discussions on science. She was using the question-asking technique, and the children were responding with great reluctance. When we discussed what she was trying to achieve, she presented several goals; but it became apparent that the only one of these for which this technique was appropriate was that of finding out if the children knew the material that had been presented. However, oral questioning permitted her to find out only about the one child answering the question. She decided that it was better to get the information through written work, which would be both more informative to her and less embarrassing to the children.

Another teacher after such a discussion reexamined her

approach to her class's social studies discussion group. She realized that her major purpose in asking questions was not to find out if the children knew the material that had been presented (i.e., the teacher's answers), but to teach them to engage in discussion. She had been troubled that this lesson was always competitive, usually filled with nasty comments, and often led to some of the children feeling bad that others were brighter. She was able to change the tone of the lesson dramatically by beginning to ask questions to which she did not know the answers. To insure that all participants would have answers to contribute, before the meeting of the discussion group she would give each child different material pertaining to the discussion. A competitive lesson was thereby changed into an informative, pleasurable discussion time.

Another teacher had been teaching a biological science course with a good deal of success to a group of disturbed children. When she got to the lesson on insects, the class suddenly became chaotic. In describing what she had done with that lesson, she said that since she knew that the children had some anxieties about insects she had decided to bring the bugs into the class and first talk with the children about their anxieties. Until this point she had only talked about anxieties if a child had brought up a particular issue; otherwise she had tried to deal with the things that might perturb them in the context of the lesson. For example, if a disease was discussed, she would be sure to include the cure of the disease, the way to avoid contracting it, and, without directly saying so, the indications that the children in the group did not have the disease. In this lesson about insects her goal had changed; it was to encourage the experience of feelings about bugs, rather than the understanding of bugs. Anxiety is not the only feeling children have about bugs. Most boys, for example, when confronted by a flying bug have an almost overwhelming desire to chase it. With the real bugs present, these real feelings were stimulated. Reading about bugs and seeing pictures of them also can stimulate both anxiety and excitement, but at an intellectual level where the anxiety and excitement are not at all intense and can be contained fairly easily, so that learning can take place.

This incident can be explained in terms of psychic structure.

The children certainly had anxieties about insects and other issues studied in biology. The structure of the class study provided them with ego support and helped contain their anxiety, while helping them to develop ways of dealing with the anxieties by learning. Furthermore, the intellectual approach to the subject matter kept them at some distance from their anxiety. When the teacher said, "Today we are going to discuss what scares you about insects," and, in addition, stimulated both anxiety and excitement *in reality,* all the support was gone and chaos ensued.

In the meeting the psychic aspect of the incident was discussed, but most important to the teacher was the issue of maintaining her goal of teaching about the subject matter. It was a goal that had been chosen because of the value to the children in learning about biology, which deals with many significant issues that a child can learn about at a distance. The biological functions of animals, for example, are fascinating to every child because of their similarity to the functions of man, but they arouse less anxiety in an anxious child because animals are not human. The value of this distance is lost when a real experience is brought in, since more feelings are stimulated and learning is then impeded.

In the selection of goals, and of the materials to achieve them, many aspects (cognitive, subject matter, etc.) are usually considered. It is also important to consider the psychological issues involved (more fully discussed in the next chapter). At one time I attempted to develop a set of criteria for selecting psychologically appropriate material for beginning readers, which I believed would be helpful to the classroom teacher. However, we discovered that such guidelines have only limited value, unless the teacher applying them has a thorough understanding of the psychological issues involved. We gave three teachers a series of statements based on assumptions derived from psychoanalytic theory, to use in rating some beginning reading books. They were to proceed in the following manner: they were to assume the statements were accurate; they were to rate each book + or − for each statement, to indicate whether the book had the element described in the statement; and then they were to give an overall rating based on the statements. It happened that the book the teachers disliked most, the most common basal reader, met more of the criteria than the other books. That is, the most typical Dick and Jane reader was the most psychologically sound of the selection. Two of the three teachers gave a lower overall rating to this book than the others, even though if they had added up the number of + ratings, it would have come out highest. Only the teacher who had previously worked with a psychoanalytically oriented instructor, and understood some of the process by which the criteria had been derived, could give an accurate overall judgement. The other teachers' inner bias (undoubtedly influenced by current criticism of basal readers) was so strong that it overcame the statements of the criterial rating sheet. These results reaffirmed that in teaching teachers it is not enough to indicate rules or guidelines for selection. The teachers have to experience and understand the process whereby the guidelines are established.

In developing individual curricula at the Orthogenic School, we first ask what the child's psychological needs are. We then try to review the spectrum of subject matter to see what would best fill these needs. For example, one very bright boy could solve distant intellectual problems very easily, but was not able to see the reality before him clearly. We chose for him a botany course that required the copying of plants and other nature forms, to give him experience with a neutral closeness that might be beneficial in developing the ability to look at less neutral closeness. Another boy had leaning toward transvestitism, which we speculated was a manifestation of an extreme curiosity about women and an effort to master it. We selected for his literature course books that contained very good and perceptive characterizations of women.

In the setting of the Orthogenic School it is possible to plan individual courses of study, since the classes are small and the teachers have enough depth of knowledge about each student to answer the question, "What does this child need?" This kind of planning does not determine the entire curriculum, of course. We also consider the child's cognitive development, the demands of society, and the academic interests of the teachers. However, questions about the needs of each child can lead to the planning of courses of study that are psychologically helpful and to the avoidance of those that are likely to be unnecessarily psychologically difficult. This kind of question can be asked when planning a curriculum for a whole class of children, with reference to expectable psychological needs at various levels. Student teachers at the nursery school asked this question about a group of four- and five-year-olds. Observing their fascination with vehicles and the pace of their locomotion and knowing the importance of successful initiative at this phase of psychosocial development, the teachers designed a unit on the mastery of speed.

Another area that could benefit from consideration of psychological needs is reading, at all levels. A review of high school reading lists makes it apparent that compilers would do well to attend to the psychological structure of teenagers, as well as to their intellectual competence. At times, a bright student is not able to grasp an issue because it is at variance with the student's emotional development, or is able to grasp it only at emotional cost. For example, an adolescent boy was asked to compare the old story of Cinderella with the Walt Disney version. The teacher was trying to demonstrate that the old tale, with its violent punishment for the sisters, was sounder psychologically than the modern tale because of the extreme clarity of the issues presented. The boy, however, came to the opposite conclusion. He concluded that they both had the same morality, but that the old one "comes off like the nineteenth-century Billy Jack"; that the author of the original was more interested in violence than subtlety. The boy himself used violent talk and showed interest in television shows containing a great deal of violence shown in a farcical fashion. While the teacher may have been accurate in her assessment of the relative psychological merit of the two fairy tales for five- and six-year-olds, she seemed not to have considered how useful psychologically it was for a sixteen-year-old. Since he had not yet fully mastered and integrated his own violent feelings, he could not understand how anything violent could be didactically sound for a younger child.

Though I have long been intensely interested in and involved with education, I have never myself been a classroom teacher. Over the years of classroom observation and interchange with teachers reflected in this chapter, it has been remarkably and repeatedly evident to me that while to be an understanding person is hard enough, to be an understanding teacher is a master art.

SIX

Attracting the Attention
of the Inattentive
(A First Step to Learning)

Many children who come to us suffer from what is called attention deficit disorder. It is manifest in the classroom by the child not being able to pay attention for any sustained period to what the teacher wants to teach and being very easily distracted. The problem is perhaps one of paying some attention to too many things, and thus not being able to pay adequate attention to any. Other of our children are called autistic-like. This disorder is also manifest in the classroom by the child not paying attention to what the teacher wants to teach, and by not seeming interested in anything at all. The problem is perhaps one of paying too much attention to internal stimulation and thus not being able to pay adequate attention to external stimulation. Attention deficit and autistic-like disorders are two of many that lead to youngsters being inattentive. Being able to capture and hold the attention of students is a critical factor in teaching.

The first striking example of this principle for me occurred when I was a counselor responsible for a group of boys, most of whom could not yet read. At the time I was taking courses in remedial reading and was practicing on my charges the skills and principles I was learning. I was unsuccessful in teaching three of these boys until we somehow hit upon reading material that captured their attention. One boy found a book about the alphabet that he insisted on reading himself, another was intrigued by reading signs, and the third learned by writing swear words. Prior to these finds all three had been highly motivated to learn to read and had seemed to struggle to do so. They had all been in an intellectual atmosphere, surrounded by stimulating reading material and had been given books that were directed at their interests. But even this combination of conditions had not led to their being able to learn. Once their attention was captured by the material itself, the principles and skills I had learned in those remedial reading courses became invaluable. We tried to understand what it was about the material that so attracted each of them, and with intimate knowledge of their life histories, we could make some speculations. The boy who learned by reading signs had twice had to have his stomach pumped because he had taken overdoses of aspirin. He had subsequently explained that he had taken the aspirin because he knew that taking a little aspirin made him feel better, so he had reasoned that taking a lot would make him feel much better. We speculated that he might have believed that if he had been able to read the warning sign he would have known of the danger and known not to take the aspirin; thus, it had become critically important to him to know what signs meant. For the boy who learned by writing swear words, the issues of self-control and expression of aggression were of paramount importance. He was struggling in his life to find a way of expressing his anger that would not prove to be destructive or bring criticism upon himself. By writing swear words, the unacceptable could become highly valued. Though I would not let him swear at me generally, I was always pleased at his writing.

Our experiences of this variety have been supported by the experiences of other educators, like Sylvia Ashton-Warner, who were able to teach reading to difficult pupils by using emotionally significant subject matter.[1] Some remedial reading teachers have used the child's own stories to teach reading, and some beginning reading teachers have used the "experience" method of teaching, whereby the group of children create reading material by recounting their own experiences.

It seemed to me that if we could extract the underlying explanation from these experiences, it might be possible to develop some broad principles that would enable us to select subject matter more likely to attract the attention of students and, thus, to facilitate their learning. For those children, at the Orthogenic School or anywhere else, who suffer from attentional difficulties, material that can engage and keep attention can be invaluable to learning. David Rapaport's theory of attention cathexis suggests a possible explanation.[2] From that theory it can be deduced that material related to the "psychic striving" of an individual is more likely to be attended to and that knowledge of an individual's psyche can help in selection of attention-attracting material. Rapaport's theory further suggests that theories of typical psychic development can give indication of specific areas that would be attractive to children at various stages of development, inasmuch as such theories (as Anna Freud's,[3] Lili Peller's,[4] and Erik Erikson's[5]) delineate the typical psychic striving at various stages of development. Of course, good teachers know without theory that certain subject matter is attractive at particular ages, and make use of this knowledge to enhance learning. For example, a first grade teacher I knew would have her whole class fascinated every year with a unit on dinosaurs. Commercial companies profit from knowledge of this same age-related appeal by manufacturing models of prehistoric creatures in a variety of sizes and materials. It is interesting to try to understand why three- to six-year-olds can become so intrigued with dinosaurs. Is it the power of the (like them) developmentally unsophisticated creatures? Or is it the thick skin, spikes and other wonders shielding the (like them) vulnerable? Or is it the resemblance to the creatures of their dreams or some other symbolism that makes the dinosaurs so fascinating? I don't know a definitive explanation, and continue to be amazed by certain youngsters' ability to pronounce (and sometimes even spell) such monstrosities as "Tyrannosaurus rex."

In my meetings with the teachers of the Orthogenic School, I have tried to incorporate these principles as we have selected material and developed curricula for the children. Some of the results of these efforts have been earlier described. The principles have never been pure, and it has always been difficult to keep track of exactly what we did. We have always been much too busy. I have had hopes of producing material that could be of use in other settings with other children whose attention it was also difficult to attract. Since those hopes have not yet been realized, I will herein provide the principles in lieu of the product. Since reading is such a basic skill for becoming educated, and since I have long been interested in that area, I will suggest as exemplars some principles specific to the stage of development when reading is typically taught. I will also describe some of our experience with a science curriculum that we developed and used in a (somewhat more than usual, for us) controlled and recorded setting.

According to my understanding of Rapaport, we all have a limited amount of psychic energy for the specific purpose of conscious awareness. This type of energy is called attention cathexis. Various excitations, both inside our psyche and in the world around us, compete with each other to attract this limited amount of energy. Those that win out are the ones that become conscious. That is, we are not automatically aware (conscious) of every stimulation that impinges on us, but only of those that manage to attract this special psychic energy. I could sleep through a thunderstorm or train whistle, but not through the whimpering of my infant son.

It is also an assumption of the theory that states of anxiety and other states of acute defense diminish the amount of attention cathexis available. The more anxious we are, the less energy we have available for attending, for becoming aware of stimuli. This assumption is generally corroborated by the common observation that when children are exceedingly anxious they cannot pay attention and cannot learn. I believe that almost everyone has had the experience, either as teacher, pupil, or observer, of the frightened child who is unable to think or answer at all because of tension about giving an answer. Relating this principle to the content of readers, we can assume that the more anxiety-provoking the content, the less energy the child will have available for awareness of stimuli, the less likely the child will be to become conscious of the words subsequently presented and, therefore, the less likely the child will be to learn to read. In general, any time the curiculum arouses extreme anxiety, energy will be needed to contend with it, and students will not have the psychic energy available to attend to the learning task—unless the learning task itself reduces that anxiety. Of course, a continuing problem is that most drive or motive-relevant subjects have some anxiety connected to them. Optimum material is not free from issues that arouse anxiety, but free from issues that arouse consuming or debilitating anxiety.

Assuming that the learner has available a reservoir of energy for the attention cathexis "pool," the question then is: What are the laws governing the movement of this psychic energy? (What are the factors that determine to what we pay attention?) Rapaport suggests a number of them, some of which are incorporated in most beginning reading programs and in most teaching strategies. One such factor is novelty. In the following discussion I will be elaborating only on those determining factors that are not as commonly incorporated.

According to Rapaport's theory, other factors being equal, stimuli that are related to drives or other motives are likely to attract attention cathexis proportionate to the strength of the motivation. One is more likely to be aware of stimuli that are related to strong motivation. There is, of course, the exception that motives that are strongly defended against (counter-cathected) will not attract this cathexis. That is, food is generally highly cathected, but also counter-cathected to the extent that one is worried about such things as obesity and cholesterol as detrimental to attractiveness and health. This can mean that when one is hungry, the first thing one sees in a department store is the candy counter or, in a book, words relating to food. However, if one has strong inhibitions against eating sweets, one might walk past the candy counter without noticing it, and misread words related to candy.

Rapaport further indicates that excitations related to drive-derivatives as well as to drives will, all things being equal, attract attention cathexis (the stronger, the more likely to attract). Drive-derivatives can be seen as those desires that are outgrowths of drives, covering most of what one might think of as having any emotional charge. If we look at the drive development of a person at various ages and at the structural development at those ages, we can speculate as to what the drive-derivatives might typically be and what would be likely to have an emotional charge. To exemplify this process, the following is a consideration of the psychic status of the child at the usual age of beginning to read, with some speculation as to the implications for the kind of material that would be likely to attract that child's attention. To understand what will be attention-attracting to a person, one has to understand the person's structure—not just what the person wants, but the conflicts about what that person wants, and the nature and relative strengths of the forces operating. For example, one might expect that adolescents would consistently be intrigued by material related to sex. However, over this past century there has been a great change in societal attitudes toward adolescent sexuality. Whether, and to what degree, the inhibitions surrounding sex would lead to feelings of guilt and, therefore, inability to attend to the material, has varied from decade to decade. Sexual material that a few decades ago would have been likely to arouse in typical middle class youngsters such inhibiting guilt that they would not look at it, is viewed openly today.

I have selected the theories of Erik Erikson, Anna Freud, and Lili Peller from which to derive ideas of what would be likely to attract the attention of a more or less typical seven-year-old, because each of them has very specifically discussed stages of development from an ego psychological point of view. They each integrate the elements that Rapaport points to as being important in determining what would typically be most likely to attract attention cathexis at particular ages.

As discussed in an earlier chapter, the age of learning to read comes at the beginning of what Erikson calls the stage of industry versus inferiority. This stage can be related to the resolution of the Oedipal conflict. In a successful resolution, the child gives up the desire for the parent of the opposite sex by identifying with the parent of the same sex. The child begins to turn to sources of gratification other than the family in order to gain more distance from the conflicts of competition for parental love. The child thus enters the social world and begins to acquire its tools.

In this context, it would seem that material about the family would be counter-indicated for children at this age. Theoretically, the family represents a conflict that the healthy child is just mastering. The experience of going out to school can offer some relief from it. Material that would arouse it would require more energy to cope with and would leave less energy for learning. The healthy child's engagement in a process of seeking gratification in the social sphere and identification with the work world would also indicate that the psychic organization would be better served by material that is oriented away from the family.

ATTRACTING THE ATTENTION OF THE INATTENTIVE

Anna Freud considered the level of psychological achievement of a child at any given point to be a result of the interaction among three areas: drive development, structural development (ego-superego), and environmental influences. In
other words, it is a result of maturation (drive development),
structuralization (ego-superego development), and adaptation (reaction to environment). She traced this kind of
development in several areas, calling these courses "developmental lines." The lines she presented were not considered to
be exhaustive of all possible lines of development, and I will
use only three of those suggested by her: from "dependency to
emotional self-reliance and adult object relations"; "from
suckling to rational eating"; and "from the body to the toy and
from play to work."[6]

In the line of development from "dependency to emotional
self-reliance and adult object relations," she, too, indicates
that in latency-age development the libidinal investment is
away from the parental figures to contemporaries, community
groups, teachers, and leaders. The line of growth is gradually
from dependence to independence, with the change in focus
of relationships away from the family. Her analysis also indicates that reading material with subject matter other than
family would be ego-syntonic. As part of this growth toward
independence, impersonal ideals and aim-inhibited sublimated interests develop. This development would explain the
attraction of the "good versus bad" theme of cowboys and
Indians, or superheroes, as impersonal ideals, and the attraction of dinosaurs or fire trucks as aim-inhibited sublimated
interests. Such topics generally seem to be more commercially
than educationally exploited.

In regard to the line "from suckling to rational eating," she
postulates that at latency the interest in food is desexualized,
and pleasure in eating, if anything, is increased. Attitudes
toward food and eating become more rational. Since the interest in food is drive-related, and pleasure in eating might be
increased, material about food and eating is ego-syntonic. The
combination of increase in rational attitudes toward food with
increase in pleasure derived from it would seem to make anything related to food a marvelous topic for this age group.

Many alphabet books seem to be based on this principle, and some successful early science programs have the attractive base of learning about food.

The hallmark of development at this age along the line "from the body to the toy and from play to work" is the ability to modify the impulses (such as to throw, take apart, mess, hoard) and to use them positively and constructively (such as to build, plan, learn, share). When I was a counselor, the boys at this stage of development seemed to be endlessly intrigued with the stories about "Little Eddie" written by Carolyn Haywood, who managed to incorporate such themes in many of those stories.[7]

Lili Peller's particular focus is on play, which she views as the ego's attempt to deal with pressures of reality, id and superego.[8] Play is the interaction of libidinal and ego development, of drive and structure formation. She says, "For the preschool child, members of his immediate family are the hub of his emotional world. At the age of five and six he seeks in various ways release from these attachments which have caused him so many painful disappointments. He turns to the fantasies of the family romance and also to . . ."[9] Thus, one can again draw the conclusion that for the youngster who is beginning to learn to read, material about the family would make the task more difficult. Peller describes the meaning of the "family romance" that comes into importance because of this turning away from the family. It refers to the fantasy that one's parents are not one's real parents. One might think of the appeal of the Superman story in this regard; he came from another planet and was raised by parents who were not his own. This fantasy can generate an interest in faraway places (the search for the real family). It can lead to the fantasy of getting along without parents, a la Robinson Crusoe. The importance of twin stories is that with an alter ego, one does not need parents. This kind of theme is ego-syntonic for the child and, therefore, when incorporated in beginning reading material, would be more likely to attract the latency child's attention.

Peller also postulates that in the early postoedipal years anal sublimations appear on a higher level. This suggests some expressions of drive-derivatives that might intrigue the seven-year-old—that is, material expressing anal sublimation, like secrets, hiding, or hoarding. It also suggests the importance and attractiveness of accumulating facts, which can be put to use in such things as word cards and repetitive learning of details.

In explaining the stage of development of the child of about six, Peller states that the underlying anxiety is that of being alone against threatening authority. In order to compensate for this, the child becomes one of many peers—and is, therefore, not alone. This explains the significance at this age of organized games where the interaction, and being one with one's peers, are of prime importance. Rules in this context become very important, and the child begins interest in codes. To support this way of coping, material that concentrates on groups of children—peer solidarity—would be appropriate. Since the underlying anxiety is that of being alone against authority, stories of one child and an adult would be threatening and, therefore, counterindicated.

The foregoing has been suggestive of a way that content for beginning reading material can be developed or chosen, in order to draw that kind of attentiveness that enables one to concentrate and thereby begin to learn. While there are many kinds of motivation that are effective in getting the learner to attend to a learning task, including external rewards and punishment, I believe that the motivation of the intrinsic psychological appeal of the material is of particular importance at the beginning of learning and for those who have difficulty in learning.

Throughout my years as Director of the Orthogenic School, I would meet regularly with the teachers to design both individual and group curricula that were based on the principles that I have been presenting. The curricula and materials for individuals would incorporate our knowledge of the particular youngster, and the group curricula would incorporate our knowledge of the general developmental level of the group. I do not want to give the impression that all of what we used was designed by us: it was, in fact, only a small percentage. Not only does it take a great deal of time to figure out what would be psychologically appropriate, but also it is extremely difficult to incorporate the orderly progression of skills and

108

knowledge which the learners need. We would aim for designing one course a year for a class; for particular students, we would concentrate on designing material for those students who might be particularly problematic. In general we would try to make use of these principles in the selection of already available curricula and material.

Our reasoning seemed to be successful. One teacher aroused her class's enthusiasm for American history by interweaving it with their personal histories. She had each class member responsible for the period in which the student's family first came to the United States. Additionally, each student described the conditions of the family's coming. The project sometimes required contacting family members. We were not entirely certain whether conflictual issues around the families might interfere with this process. We speculated that the distance from anything personal, since it was all ancestral, would allow for the positive cathexis to be dominant. Furthermore, since these were mostly older students who were engaged in the process of trying to understand and master their pasts, we thought that the effort would be ego-syntonic.

At another time, we were having a lot of trouble with our early adolescent boys who were, literally, running around the school, getting into places where they were not supposed to be but which had obvious appeal, because of the very fact of being forbidden. We reasoned that the boys had a drive for physical discharge and a drive-derivative for finding out secrets. A rigorous physical education program could speak to the former and a good laboratory science program could speak to the latter. We were fortunate enough to find a male teacher who was competent in the areas of both physical education and science. While the new program did not entirely solve our problem, it was a significant component of the solution.

In an effort to be more systematic in our attempts to develop this kind of curriculum, we organized two classes in a somewhat different way. As described earlier, our classroom groups basically stay with their teachers throughout the day. The teacher's ability to teach is closely related to the knowledge of and relationship with each student. We therefore are often able to have a group of youngsters together who, without the teacher's support, would be unmanageable. The material presented is only one of many components in the total educational milieu. In our regular setting we have not been able to keep track of exactly what the teacher does, or the effect on the students of the material presented. We decided that if we had a teacher who taught a very limited number of classes, that teacher could have time to take notes and we could see more clearly what happened. The teacher would not have the benefit of the ongoing relationship that the regular teachers had, and the class, therefore, would be much more difficult to manage. We formed two groups of five, one with an age range of nine to thirteen, and the other with an age range of fifteen to eighteen. The younger group met three times a week for thirty minutes each time. The older group met twice a week for forty-five minutes each time. The reading and writing skills within each group were fairly disparate, but close enough to enable all the members of the class to use the same material. More important for the problem that we wanted to address, we thought that the students in each group were at a similar level of psychosexual and psychosocial development.

I have referred briefly to our experience with the older group in chapter 4. Of the five in the younger group, three were considered to be the biggest management problems in the School. Since the psychic energy of this cohort was focused on very similar issues which aroused anxiety in all of them, and since their structural development was similarly weak, the nature of their interaction was typically explosive. They would focus on similar things, get upset by similar things, and deal with their anxiety in similar acting-out kinds of ways. We tried to design a curriculum that would address exactly those issues that attracted the interest of all of them, but in a way that would lead toward constructive mastery rather than destructive acting out. For these five youngsters we thought that the dominant psychic issues were those of nurturance, aggression, and bodily function (mostly anal and sexual). This focus was related partly to their stage of psychosocial development and partly to their individual histories. We decided to design for them an animals study curriculum, because we have found that the study of animals is often a very useful way to deal with the kind of primitive issues that both fascinated and troubled them. A direct discussion of such issues can arouse too much anxiety when a youngster is at a stage of development out of it or when it is conflict-related. For example, when growing toward independence, for a youngster to avoid talking about nurturant needs is often a healthy device, protecting against the strong arousal of such needs. The study of an animal baby permits some distance and, therefore, the possibility of vicarious gratification, with emotional protection from too much need-stimulation. Similarly, one can be fascinated by the elimination process in animals without confessing that one is bewildered about one's own.

After the first year, we were satisfied that our experience with this class supported our notion that the use of such an approach facilitates both management of difficult children and learning. Though there were many incidents of disruptive behavior, the class had functioned well enough for the group to develop a sense of camaraderie, for the children to learn, and for others to request a similar class. This was no mean achievement for a group of five "unmanageable" youngsters, meeting for a relatively short amount of time with a teacher who could not know them as well as their regular teacher or have the advantage of a continuing relationship.

In order to be able to examine the specific components of the curriculum and the specific reactions of the students, the teacher took process notes after each class, and we afterwards went over them.[10] The group's study of animals was organized according to some of the usual curricular principles. That is, the scientific hierarchy of phyla was presented in order, from the sponges through the mammals, from the simplest to the most complex. The students learned about the structure of the different animals and how it was used to enable the animal to perform those necessary and fascinating functions of eating, eliminating, reproducing, escaping, and so forth. The organization of the curriculum was, thus, both scientifically sound and related to what we thought was "motive-relevant." The instructor was an experienced teacher and curriculum specialist and so used a wide variety of teaching techniques, material, and media.

We reviewed the lessons, including both lesson plans and what had actually been presented, and were able to divide them into the following five thematic categories: (1) wild animals with people, (2) dangerousness, (3) growth and development, (4) structure and function/evolution, and (5) generalized or nonanimal activity. We also reviewed the notes the teacher had taken about the class response and divided them with respect to the degree of attentiveness the youngsters gave to the lesson. There were times when the students were a delightful, eager class, asking questions and volunteering the names of esoteric classifications. There were other times when they were hellions, teasing each other nonstop, tearing up their material, disrupting, jumping in the garbage can. In our review of the notes, we tried to sort out the source of such behavior, so that we did not mistake preholiday anxiety or anxiety created by an event in the life of the School for that created by the curriculum. We were not surprised to find that the lessons that fell into one of the first three thematic categories were better and more enthusiastically attended to than those in the last two categories. It was very impressive to see these youngsters, who were often described as wild, and seemed completely uncaring of others, quietly entranced while watching, hearing, or studying about the care and nurturing of wild animals. It seemed that these children, who had such difficulty in taming their own impulses and who felt so unacceptable, while yearning to be accepted, identified with the untamed animals and thus were fascinated by seeing them nurtured, loved, and tamed. A movie that showed people engaged in the scientific study of animals, even for very benevolent purposes, was not nearly as attractive as one that showed people caring for them.

The issues of dangerousness, nurturance, elimination, and sex consistently aroused intense interest and attention. However, there were times that the interest drew attention away from the lesson rather than toward it, and engendered very disruptive behavior. Such an incident was provoked by a film on predator-prey relationships, which showed a female insect imitating the mating flash of a female firefly in order to lure the male firefly as prey. The students called the female insect a vamp, and three of the youngsters began to provoke and scapegoat a fourth. It seemed that when a dangerous animal was presented in such a way that an identification with that animal would help the students to feel strong and powerful, the lesson was attended to. However, when such an identification would make them feel threatened, anxiety would drive them to behavior that would divert them from the threatening lesson, and make them feel stronger.

While generally the lessons devoted to structure and function were less well attended to, it frequently was the case that they would evoke attention to those basic issues we thought to be of importance to these students. That attention, while intense, would be away from the lesson being presented. Members of the group would engage vigorously in making anal or sexual sounds and gestures, which stimulated mutual arousal, glee, and what many teachers call "on the ceiling" or "off the wall" behavior. Often it seemed that the cause was that the presentation was straightforward and aroused only the anxiety about the issue, without stimulating any protective, reassuring devices or defenses. For example, a youngster with a history of very early neglect and abuse could not tolerate viewing a filmstrip that, in discussing the differences between the primitive orders of mammals, compared the orders in terms of the mammary glands, nursing, and the development of the young. On the other hand, the same student was very attentive to those films that depicted a person adopting a baby animal and caring for it.

Another time, in the context of studying the evolutionary significance of amphibians and their adaptations to living on the land, a filmstrip was shown. When it noted that amphibians have no sperm-conducting organ with which to fertilize eggs, and are thus dependent on the water for this function, the group became completely chaotic. The anxieties about not having a sperm-conducting organ and about eggs being left unprotected in water were just too much to contend with. In retrospect, we realized that the teacher either should have excised this section, if it was not vital to the goals of the lesson, or prepared the class with some kind of reassurance about human development out of this state.

Many issues that are highly evocative of anxiety can be addressed in an empathic way that can bring students' attentiveness to a lesson. Two films were presented dealing with urination. In one, about scientists studying urine in order to understand territoriality, the scientists were shown smelling the animals' urine. The class reacted very negatively. They couldn't understand why the scientists were interested and how they could tolerate smelling the urine. They thought it was disgusting and sick! Another movie, also concerned with territoriality, showed a wolf marking his territory with his urine. The man in the film, desiring to become acquainted with wolf habits, then marked his territory with his urine. The students were fascinated with this film. It seemed that whether interest or anxiety would be the predominant reaction depended on the context of the presentation. Our speculation was that the critical factor was acceptance. If we assumed that the students identified with the animal, we could see that as a result of the first film they would feel less than human, since they had to be studied and examined to be understood, while as a result of the second film they would feel quite human. The first film depicted the adult being interested in studying a phenomenon that was foreign. Though the interest was positive, such an approach made the phenomenon distant and different. The second man treated the phenomenon as one that he could understand through his own experience, and thus made it close and similar.

I would say that what seemed to be the most attention-cathecting theme, on the basis of the responses of these students to the curricular content, was acceptance. For this group, characteristically hard to manage and understand, it would seem that their need to feel accepted, in the face of feeling so strange and unacceptable, was stronger than any of the psychosexual or psychosocial indicators. A frequent interaction between the class and the teacher illustrated this need and her unwitting provision for it. One of the first lessons she taught was about the barnacle, a creature with a hard-shelled exterior but a soft inside. One of its most outstanding characteristics, to people, is that it is a nuisance. The barnacle is also bizarre, as it stands on its head and waves food into its mouth with its feet. The class made a big to-do about the foolishness of the teacher for being interested in such an unattractive creature. The barnacle became a class joke, with which the teacher was frequently and affectionately teased—that she could care about such a nuisance.

SEVEN

Rebecca and How She Learned to Read

Before I knew anything of the Orthogenic School, Freud, psychoanalytic theory, or disturbed children, I had an investment in the power of learning. This is likely to have come from a Jewish heritage, through a mother who always told me to learn because knowledge was something that no one could ever take away from me. This might be why I have been particularly fascinated with those children who, having obviously powerful intellectual abilities, are nonetheless helpless in the face of life. Our successful work with such youngsters depends very much on the integration of dormitory and classroom, and on the mutually supportive work of teacher and counselor. To exemplify this integral role of the educational enterprise in our therapeutic milieu, I will present a study that is fictional in its entirety, but real in its detail. Rebecca, to whom you will presently be introduced, is a person who never existed, but whom I have invented from a multitude of experiences with many students who really existed as a very important part of the lives of the School and its Director. I hope in this way to make use of what I have learned from them, but not to intrude on their privacy.

Rebecca, who might have come to us at the age of eight, manifested a dramatic contrast between a highly developed, active mind and a helpless, inactive body. Her mind and body seemed to function separately, as though in two encapsulated universes. Since she had not joined the two together and hence was not a "person," her mind had achieved a high level of development only in isolated areas which did not relate directly to herself, or to her life's problems. She could think logically and well only about problems such as ancient history and dinosaurs that did not involve her own observation. The more distant a problem was from her life, the better she could cope with it. At the same time, since she could not recognize or accept the importance of her body, she had been able to develop neither fine nor gross body skills, like dressing herself, and sought to achieve neither. Despite a demonstrably high intellectual endowment and despite an intense intellectual interest, she had not mastered any of the normal learning tasks of an eight-year-old; she had not even begun to learn to read.

Rebecca arrived at the Orthogenic School with the essential ingredients of an exceptionally capable human being—an attractive body and a superior mind—but was painfully unable to put either to good use. Her mind was active and free so long as its gears never connected with the problems of her life. When not lost in an autistic-like reverie, she would talk on as long as anyone would listen. Though she talked with a babyish lisp, her vocabulary was excellent.

Her first encounter with the staff of the School was with me in my office. At this first meeting I have always tried to convey to my young candidate for admission a sense of the task of the School. I try to be direct about the enormity of the problem and about our willingness to address and provide help with it. In this way I am able to let the person know that we are deeply interested in forming a therapeutic alliance and to discover if it is possible to do so. Older candidates are often able in this meeting to concisely identify their most critical problem and to acknowledge their desire to get help with it. Of course, most frequently the adolescent who in my office has revealed a desperate desire to feel adequate, competent, and lovable, and who is deeply concerned about hallucinatory episodes and suicidal thoughts, will shortly after enrollment in the School become arrogant, critical, and somewhat delinquent. Nonetheless, the ability of that adolescent, even for a short period, to trust another, to be vulnerable, and to make a contract, in a sense, to engage in the struggle for health, is a sound basis for a therapeutic alliance.

Though younger children are not as able to articulate the painfulness of their psychic state, they are as aware of it as their older fellows. It is equally important to be clear to them about the therapeutic contract. It also has to be very clear to them that it is only because of drastic need that they are being separated from their parents. Only with this awareness is the separation tolerable to child and parent. (As one parent put it, the pain of being separated from her child for a year was nothing compared to the pain of watching him fail to develop.)

On Rebecca's first visit she presented the problem of mind/body separation dramatically. There she sat, trying desperately to impress me with her historical knowledge and with the seriousness of her intention to become an eminent researcher, while her inability to unwrap a piece of candy bespoke her helplessness. I neither commiserated with her about the helplessness of her body, nor became captivated by her mind (which would have been fairly easy, because what she said was extremely interesting), but rather asked her how she could become a historian if she could not read. She countered by stressing her supersensitivity when compared to other children and her consuming intellectual interest, which prevented her from being bothered with such ordinary tasks.

It was of crucial importance to let her know from the start that our efforts would be to offer gratifications of her basic needs (so candy was provided), and to help her with the mastery of those basic problems that prevented her from accomplishing the normal living tasks of an eight-year-old, such as learning to read. Furthermore, we wanted her to know that we would be acting neither because she was so very bright, nor because she was such an inadequate baby, but because she was *she*, and because what was provided was what *she* needed most.

With many of our children, it is important not to be excessive in trying to satisfy basic, primitive needs, lest the efforts be experienced as either threatening or overly seductive. I did not, therefore, offer to unwrap Rebecca's candy. (I usually like to have candy that is familiar and wrapped, to take care of some of the feelings of lack of trust that our students so frequently have, that would prevent them from trying unfamiliar food or food that might have been touched.) If we invite too much experiencing of infantile gratification, a child is in danger of becoming bound to that mode. This is an issue that requires a sensitive balance not only at the beginning of our treatment, but progressively through it. A given quantity of gratification, that is at one moment not enough, at another stage of development is just the right amount, and at another stage is too much. While it is difficult enough for parents to gauge this in normal development (When is the right time to give up the bottle?), it is even more difficult in work with our young people, whose developmental needs are often disconnected from any kind of age norms. It is important to know when that which by ordinary standards is too much, for a particular individual is not enough: when the latency-age child, though having the capability to do without, really needs help in getting dressed. It is equally important to know when that which, by that particular individual's standards, has been enough, suddenly becomes too much, when the help becomes an impediment to independent growth rather than the sustenance that permits it.

Since it is a complete change in their physical and emotional environment, coming to the Orthogenic School is for all children a highly charged event. While some children can experience it immediately as a great relief, others are threatened by the newness. How each child deals with it reflects characteristics of both personality and disturbance. Some concentrate on orienting themselves in their physical environment, others bemoan the loss of the old. Quite a few derive some comfort from physical pleasure, such as eating, while others are unable to eat anything.

The child with autistic tendencies is likely to fall back on an autistic defense and turn away from the onslaught of emotional experiences. Thus Rebecca's first effort to comfort herself the first evening in her dormitory was by listening to a record that she had brought with her and thereby blotting out the emotional world around her. Her counselors made many efforts to join her. When one counselor talked with her through the teddy bear that had been given her as a welcome present, she haughtily explained that she could not be tricked into thinking that her teddy bear was alive, and that she could tell that it really wasn't because it had neither nerves nor feelings. Her intellect told her that this was a stuffed animal; it did not tell her that this was obvious to one and all, and that the counselor was engaged in make-believe.

In all instances she would use her intellectual knowledge and powers of reasoning where the normal child would respond to the emotional situation. These powers would fail her because they did not permit reaching emotional decision. She could not use her great intellect to solve such problems as finding her slippers or putting them on the right feet. She had no idea where her closet was, though it had repeatedly been shown to her as her belongings had been put into it, and though it was only a few feet from her bed. When her counselor brought her slippers from the closet, she put them on the wrong feet. When her counselor suggested that they might feel more comfortable on the other feet, she did not understand what was meant.

She would not trust adults, but she permitted another child to show the way to comfort on the first evening. A girl in the dormitory, who was a little older and had been at the School for about two years, talked with Rebecca about the night— how she could get the night counselor if she was scared, or could waken one of the other older girls in the dormitory, and how she would feel better in the morning after a good night's sleep and the coming of light. She not only talked about, but also demonstrated physically, what would happen. She brought her to the night counselor's room and stretched her arms as she would on arising next morning. With adults Rebecca could not relax her intellectual protection; that this emotional appeal came from another child made it more acceptable. Moreover, since the child spoke in the language of her emotional needs—the body and her anxiety—she could respond and finally begin to relax. Her counselor, though in line with these efforts at keeping to the immediate situation, had to pose simple problems of living as complex intellectual problems, for only then could Rebecca master them. At snack time she was unable to eat, but when the counselor told her that she had to make the very difficult, complex, and important decision of which cookie she wanted, she ate.

For those students who are able to observe others, the action around them is important in helping them to be comfortable in the initial period. Even though the transition to the School absorbs their energies, so that most seem not to be able to attend to much else, we frequently find that these initial observations have made a lasting impact. One young woman, who had come to the School at fifteen following a suicide attempt, many years later told me that though she had been very scared and frequently negative about her entry into the School, her teacher's attitude toward another child was deeply impressive and reassuring to her. The other child was severely autistic, with little speech, very unusual mannerisms, and, sometimes, violent physical outbursts. The young woman told me that the respect with which the teacher treated this child, in the face of extreme difficulty in managing and understanding him, held out to her the slim hope that she might also receive such respect and concern.

People have often asked about the effect that the presence of more seriously disturbed students has on the better-integrated students. Though the arrangement has many difficulties, the reaction of this young woman expresses most cogently its greatest value. The more severely disturbed youngsters often express the deepest fears and most-hidden anxieties of the less disturbed. The staff's acceptance of the turbulence of the most-distressed children helps the others to begin to trust that perhaps we can accept and understand them, too. When they can see some alleviation of the profound distress of these children and some amelioration of the destructive actions and bizarre behavior, they can begin to feel that perhaps there is some hope for alleviation of their own less-profound distress and amelioration of their own less-bizarre symptoms.

Rebecca quickly became dependent on us. In the morning she never arose without encouragement and help. She was never aware of time, so she would, for instance, not take any initiative in going to or getting ready for meals. For almost all of her basic needs she was dependent on her counselors, not only to help fill them, but even to be aware of them.

She was unable to use a fork or spoon, could eat only with her hands, and even that only in incredibly clumsy ways. She could barely manage to dress herself; her limp body had no muscle tone. Even the manipulative skills she possessed were those of a four-year-old. Physically she sought very infantile gratifications, laying her head in our laps and deriving sensuous pleasure from the feel of food. This acceptance of physical contact was emotionally unrelated. Since it was encapsulated, it never developed into any kind of relationship to others or to her body. When she later could afford to be aware of her reactions to such contact, she was extremely anxious about it.

In any situation presenting a problem, she consistently used only her intellect, in most abstract ways unrelated to the real problem at hand. Since she did not dare to look at the immediate situation, most likely out of fear of what she then might learn, the use of her intellect could never lead to real understanding, let alone mastery. This mechanism was, perhaps, most strikingly apparent when she made an effort to apply her intellect to something about her body. Since she was as yet unable to experience her body, the intellectual action continued to be dissociated. When she would try to get her shoes on the right feet, she could not do it by the "feel" but had to hold the shoe up to her foot to match the way the soles went. When she tried to engage in doll play, she could discuss the great need for physical contact, and even quote Harlow's experiments with monkeys; but despite many demonstrations by her older dorm mates, she was not able to hold a doll in any but the most awkward fashion.

Many of our students are able to pursue scientific abstractions with great ease but unable to think about practical or emotional issues. For some, the reason for their facility in science is related to the perceived constancy of abstraction. One boy expressed this idea after he had mastered some aspects of arithmetic but was still unable to read even a preprimer. He told us that the reason he could do math but not read was that "six is always six," and he held up his fingers to demonstrate, but an "e" is sometimes pronounced one way and sometimes another.

For many reasons, most of our children suffer from deep feelings of shame and inadequacy about their bodies. The extreme use of intellect for children like Rebecca can be a protective shelter, hiding from the world and self a body felt to be inadequate and something to be ashamed of. When Rebecca was a toddler her mother had been concerned about what she considered to be an undue amount of hair growth, which Rebecca experienced as evidence that she was strange. We speculated that her not looking at herself protected her from seeing this hair growth, but it also protected her from seeing that it did not make her unattractive.

There is no direct approach to reconstructing a self or to overcoming the anxieties that created its misdevelopment. What one can do is provide the setting conducive for and the help required by the child for such reconstruction. The first efforts in Rebecca's treatment were to teach her to play like an eight-year-old because it is through play that mind and body interact as a unit in the young child, and learn to interact in ever more complex situations. At the time the staff knew little of the dynamics of Rebecca's psyche; they came to know her psyche through Rebecca, as she came to understand and reveal herself. The gross basis for the treatment decision was simply that play is an important step in development and serves important functions. Her inability to move or use her body clearly showed that she had never had the requisite play experiences which would lead to an eight-year-old's mastery. If she could play, she could gain such mastery. By stressing play in which both mind and body were involved, the staff stayed away from emphasizing or rewarding one at the expense of the other.

Throughout her stay at the School, Rebecca was both frustrating and delightful. One source of delight was her ability to express herself so aptly. When she could turn her mind to immediate matters, she was always extremely sensitive to the staff's intentions, which she could very quickly recognize and could state explicitly—"Progress here is kind of nice because it means playing with more things." She made this statement after several months at the School, during which she had tried out the various kinds of play presented and had found her own way to make use of them. At first she was delighted with playing very simple games of chance and games such as Redlight Greenlight. In these games, she found that at last she was not expected to perform in order to win; all she had to do was turn a dial or run when no one was looking. After a while the games became a means of expressing a very crucial issue. She would become terribly upset when she lost and would cry and complain with great histrionics that the other girls were cheating. The vehemence of her response was as though to a much greater loss and seemed to be an expression of distress at life's dependence on chance, on those factors that she did not understand and could not control.

Many of our children feel that they have no control over major happenings in their lives. For Rebecca the feeling seemed related to her powerlessness over her parents' divorce and her inner conviction that her stepsister had cheated her out of her father's love. Once she had let the staff know, with her tearful carryings-on, that they must be predictable and not let her be cheated, she gave up these games of chance and began to concentrate her energies on those forms of play over which she felt she had more control. She verified our speculation that control, predictability, and positive feelings toward her were the crucial issues, when later she did go back to these games for a short period. She and her counselor played a game with a spinner involving each person's choosing a number. Far from becoming upset at a loss, she now managed to view every outcome as some kind of victory. She maintained that she could predict whose number would come up and held to her belief in her predictive powers even when she was proved wrong. Furthermore, she always reacted as though she were winning. If neither player's number was spun, she said that at least it wasn't the counselor's, and if the counselor's number came up she said that hers would the next time. Through play, she had first expressed her great distress at the unpredictability of the most important things in her life and her conviction that things could not come out right enough for her. So, similarly, through play she later could say that she was beginning to feel an ability to control her life and to be able to win at it.

It was very important during the first period that the staff simply accept her outbursts. If we had tried to fix the games' wheel of fortune in order to have peace, we would have been presenting a false world over which she still had no control, and she would have missed the opportunity for an important experience of mastery. These games were the playground where she could not only express her distress at not being able to control everything in life, but where she could also begin to accept that there are things in life over which one really has no control. Such matters are easier to accept around games than around vital events like parents' moods or separations.

It was important during the later period not to contradict her belief in her clairvoyance. Just as it would have been futile to try to convince her initially that the other children were not responsible for her bad luck, it would have been futile to try to convince her then that she could not predict the future. The prescription for both misperceptions was to facilitate her real mastery, since the ability to have real control would give her the strength to accept those areas where she really had no control. If we had embarked on such a futile enterprise, she would only have felt that we did not really understand her— either her pain at being unable to predict and control, or her pleasure that she was gradually becoming able to do so.

The areas of play where such real control can be developed are those of simple physical mastery and of fantasy. Rebecca's first choice was fantasy. Her actors were the stuffed animals which she had at first rejected. Certain aspects of the School's practice facilitated her ability to engage in that suspension of disbelief intrinsic to all fantasy, which at first had been too threatening for her. Every student upon coming to the School receives a stuffed animal. The reason for this practice can be understood if one thinks about the attributes normally attached to stuffed animals—cuddliness, warmth, comfort. These are exactly what is needed by a person entering a new and strange situation. Many animals also incorporate characteristics of strength and fierceness which make them symbolically protective. Since stuffed animals are also associated with babyishness, we usually try to incorporate sophistication in our animal gifts to our older students. Everyone also gets a stuffed animal on Christmas. The animals are made by the school seamstress with assistance from one or more staff members in the selection of patterns and material. Further assistance is rendered by the whole staff in stuffing and sewing. The animals are very highly emotionally invested by the staff when the decisions are made as to which child will get which animal. The tradition is thus a personalized affair.

On Rebecca's first Christmas she received a kangaroo with a single baby, to give, in a small way, some gratification for and acknowledgement of one of her fondest desires, to be the only one. The counselors in Rebecca's dormitory looked after the animals of the dorm with the greatest of care. Every evening they were part of the bedtime preparation. Some animals were carefully tucked in with their mistresses, while others were stationed in strategic positions to keep watch through the night. No one for a moment thought an animal was alive, but most of the girls willingly engaged in the tender suspension of disbelief that was entailed. A most clear example of the value of this use of animals occurred with my own son. He had more or less ignored the stuffed animals that he had had since birth despite my counselor-like ministrations to them. When he was almost four, we moved to another city. He spontaneously began to position his biggest animal at the outer edge of his bed and continued this practice until he was more secure with his new abode. For several years, he would when particularly anxious stand this animal in front of his bedroom door. When animals have been emotionally invested by adults, it seems that they provide the tangible reassurance and comfort to accompany the implied message, "I know that you are afraid, and though your fears in reality are unfounded, I want you to have reassurance and comfort."

The students at the Orthogenic School receive gifts on their birthdays, on the anniversaries of their coming to the School, and on several holidays. Their snacks and entertainment are generally provided. In addition, they each receive a weekly allowance. The purpose of the allowance is to enable them to buy whatever they want. The message that we encourage them to select what they themselves really want is more important than the actual selection. The things that they can buy with their allowances could not have much greater intrinsic value than many of the things they have already, since they are surrounded by desirable playthings, as part of the therapeutic effort to seduce them into life, to convince them that life can be good, and to convey to them that the staff thinks that they are worthy of the best. These possessions take on a value that in one respect far outweighs that of the most expensive gift, since the choice is entirely theirs.

With her allowance Rebecca bought a stuffed cat, apparently a symbolic replica of the cat she had had at home. She slept with and cuddled the stuffed cat, as she had often done with the real one. The cat and the bear, her welcome gift, became the major protagonists in a continuing drama. They were continually engaged in a violent struggle for the best position in the forest. Rebecca took great delight in violently acting out the struggle between the two. She would wallop the animals around with such gusto that they often became depleted of stuffing. One might speculate that the intensity of the struggle was related to the intensity of conflict imagined between her parents, or between the School and her parents. The kangaroo was the mediating party, often restoring order to the forest.

During this time she was able to acquire some greater physical competency, apparently as the result of the simple removal of secondary gains that she had received from her infantile behavior, coupled with a reduction of expectations for performance. Her classroom teacher was more interested in her developing physical manipulative skill than in academic achievement. Rebecca once complained that though her dorm mates thought she was brilliant at history, her teacher thought she was lousy at pasting.

It has often been our experience that relaxing demands in some areas produces gains in others. One graduate of the School, reflecting on his experience, felt that simple abandonment of the need for academic achievement had so much reduced his internal pressure as to account for the disappearance, within a few months of his coming to the School, of almost all signs of the tics and twitches that had beset him.

Rebecca was able to learn to jump rope, as part of the routine in her daily physical education classes with her teacher and six classmates, in which they regularly did simple exercises and played simple games. This accomplishment was very important to her, though she had never been able previously to admit how bad she felt about her physical incompetence. Even after she had this mastery fairly well secured, the former hesitancy and awkwardness would come back when her bodily anxiety was intensified, as on a day when she was to go to the dentist. She then would not be able to relax into the rhythm and timing necessary for jumping rope, and would be unable even to take her turn.

As she became more secure in her physical mastery, the nature of her play with the animals began to change. She became interested in collecting a wide variety of cats, ranging from warm and purring housecats to dangerous big cats of the jungle. It was our impression that the cats were expressions of different aspects of her personality. When she asked for a special gift of a rather expensive leopard, we agreed. She was a girl who made very few material requests, so we felt that this request had particular significance. It seemed to be an important question about our approval of her more aggressive nature and her efforts to express it. Later she told us that for her the cats were in fact very clearly representations of specific qualities. The Persian cat was intelligence; the Siamese cat, jealousy; the alley cat, aggressiveness; the Cheshire cat, joy; the mixed breed cat, love; the leopard, slyness and strength; and the lioness, who finally became queen of the forest, integration.

As her gradual freeing was taking place, it was of the utmost importance that it somehow be conveyed to Rebecca that "intellect" can approve the existence and assertions of "body." The organization of the Orthogenic School provided the ideal figure to give just that reassurance—her teacher. Rebecca was in a class with six other boys and girls and her teacher from 9:00 to 3:00 five days a week. The rest of the time she spent with the six girls in her dormitory group, together with one or another of her three counselors. All caretaking functions outside of class hours were the responsibility of her counselors. Separation of the function of the mind and the function of the body was clearly provided for in this arrangement, in both time and space. While the life of the School is set up in this way, resembling to some extent the broad features of life outside the School and creating a symbolic representation of the separation between mind and body, the teacher is by no means restricted to an isolated segment of any child's life. Through participation in staff meetings, frequent informal conversations with other staff members involved in the student's care, and constant reporting, the teacher is part of the staff's continual evaluation and reevaluation of the needs of the student and of the therapeutic direction most advisable. It is in the context of the young person's total psychological well-being that the teacher builds a curriculum for and relationship with the student.

No one who comes to the Orthogenic School is expected to do any kind of academic work until the staff has some idea of its meaning and value to that person. For Rebecca, not only would such work have reminded her of her previous school failure, but it also would have reinforced her view that the mind is only for intellectual matters.

Rebecca was placed in a class in which there was great variation in the emphasis placed on academic learning. While three of the students were engaged with academics throughout the day, for the other three the engagement was similar to Rebecca's. Her day was fairly regularly divided, so that she would know approximately what to expect each day as far as a general routine was concerned. Each morning there would be on her desk some of her favorite candies and some kind of manipulative material that had been carefully selected for her by her teacher. She might cut, paste, color, work with clay, or do absolutely nothing. The candy and manipulative material, tokens of her teacher's thought of her, would tide her over until the teacher came to spend some time with her.

Next came juice time. Until this time the students were engaged in individual activities; a common, desirable food signalled the beginning of common interests and activities. After juice time came physical education in the gym. Then the younger students joined in a circle to engage in activities involving the use of the body, particularly movement and exploration. They played various rhythm games and games like the one requiring that they identify objects by feeling them inside a box. The English and literature period for the younger students included spelling time. The children would select words to be written on the blackboard, choosing the kinds of words that they wanted to learn—for instance, categories of good, bad, or scary. The emphasis was not on learning to spell or read but on words as expressions of important feelings.

After lunch came recess time, when either group or individual activities were planned depending on the need engendered by the rhythm of the day. Activities usually involved gross body movements. The remainder of the day, while academically oriented for some, for Rebecca was allocated to projects and art. Finally there was free time, when she could do what she chose, either from her own ingenuity or the offerings of the teacher, or do nothing. Thus, the main emphasis in the pattern of Rebecca's intellectual world was on the satisfaction of physical needs and body mastery.

Reading material was at all times abundantly available in Rebecca's classroom. There were varieties of reading series as well as many interest-filled books. From time to time, Rebecca would attempt to master a book, and her teacher would offer to teach her. Though Rebecca knew the sounds of all the letters, her attempts to put them together invariably led to incomprehensible caricaturization: "gu-i-er-ul" never became "girl."

When Rebecca's body had become to some degree emotionally expressive, and when her teacher had demonstrated that her and, therefore, her mind's, purpose was first to work with her body, Rebecca could reveal some of her deepest concerns and use her mind to look at them, with her teacher.

For Rebecca, as for many children who feel that they are not able to control important aspects of their lives, it was the elimination function that was of greatest importance to master. It was around the process and product of elimination that a most important intellectual learning experience took place, a crucial experience that helped her to learn that it was safe to look at her body and body products and to examine the body issues of importance to her.

Although the children were free to use the washroom at any time, Rebecca did not do so during class time for many months. She was horrified that it was so close to the classroom, so that everyone would know that she was there and might even hear what she was doing. After months of discussion in which her teacher and other classmates assured her that the activities that took place on the toilet were common and well-known to everyone, and that the time spent by several classmates in front of the large mirror over the washbasin was time well spent, she was finally able to make use of the washroom. When she did, it was an opportunity to communicate a concern, much more than to satisfy a physical need. She would return to the classroom in a state of great anxiety that she had diarrhea. Her teacher would give the matter her immediate attention and would invariably find a perfectly normal stool. She would reassure Rebecca as to her state of health and at the same time encourage her in the expression of such concerns. She recognized that for Rebecca to talk about these matters was a tremendous achievement, for even with the other children Rebecca usually acted as though feces were to be disdained. For example, when two of the girls were giggling about "dog-doo" and "cow-doo," one of them asked Rebecca if she ever thought about "cat-doo," since the cat was her favorite animal. Rebecca replied that she had never "thought about dirty things like that." Now she was finally ready to begin to believe that things about the body could also be important, even things that she had up until this time considered "dirty."

After numerous discussions of the product—its consistency, and color, and the meaning thereof—it was time to deal with the process. When it was clear that Rebecca would consider it a support rather than an intrusion, her teacher joined her when she went to the toilet. The emotional-intellectual conversation that ensued had to be begun by the teacher. She spoke to Rebecca in two languages, that of the mind and that of the body, about the issue with which Rebecca was at that moment physically, emotionally, and intellectually involved, the defecating process. This was the beginning of months of daily sessions in the washroom, during which Rebecca could continue the conversation started by her teacher and use her mind to reflect on and help her body in the mastery of the elimination process.

She could not look at the feces because to her they were all bad. When her teacher remarked that it was curious that she never showed her "good" feces, but only the feces that she was worried about, she was much surprised. She thought that it was all the same, all waste, and it had never occurred to her that there could be "good" feces. Her ability to talk about and look at her body products developed along with her ability to talk about and look at her body. Trips to the washroom were related to the mirror and to careful examination of her face and arms, with comparisons of hair growth on her teacher and herself. She was able to let her teacher know of her concern about looking different from others. Her teacher was able to demonstrate both that the difference was less extreme than she believed it to be and that the difference that existed did not interfere with her ability to be loved.

As these important actions and interactions were taking place, Rebecca was making small degrees of progress in other bodily activities, and in reading. If she could look at her body products and her own body freely, with a lesser degree of shame, she could look at words. If she could begin to master the most important bodily process, she could begin to master other processes. The strong anxiety that had surrounded looking at and inspecting objects (her feces, numbers, letters) was at last lifting.

Once Rebecca had repeatedly had the crucial experience of using her mind to gain mastery of the elimination process and reassurance about her own physical normality and attractiveness, she was able to use it for mastery of other bodily activities. Until this time she had shown no active desire to acquire bodily skills. Those that she had, like jumping rope, had been acquired without any conscious effort. When thoughts about her body no longer made her so intensely anxious, she could pay attention to it. When she could do this, she began to want to use her body and to gain pleasure from greater physical skill. She had gained a great deal of affection and approval from her teacher, not by the intellect alone, nor by the body alone, but by the use of the two together. She knew that she need not fear loss of affection if she continued to use her mind and body together.

It was shortly after her second Easter at the School that the intermeshing of the gears of Rebecca's mind and body began to carry her forward obviously in the development of physical mastery. Holidays at the School are traditionally celebrated in such a way as to make pleasurable emotional exclamation points in the rhythm of the year. A holiday provides another occasion for making life attractive and for reasserting the staff's belief that the students are worth many good things. The great emphasis that we put on holidays makes them focal points for an orientation in time. Developing time orientation was very important for Rebecca who, when she came to the School, did not even know her birthdate. To Rebecca an important feature of a holiday was the superabundance of food. We celebrate Easter, for instance, with outstanding emphasis on the enjoyment of eating. When the children wake up they find paper "bunny tracks" leading from the doors of their dormitories to the room where their Easter baskets and presents are hidden. The use of the Easter Bunny as the giver of such gifts serves the very important function, particularly for youngsters like Rebecca, of stating that the gift is for the child to accept or reject, with no need to feel beholden to the staff or to use or like the gift in order not to hurt the staff's feelings.

It was no accident that the first physical activity on which Rebecca chose to use her intellect was one that came out of this holiday. The holidays had already made possible for her the beginning of temporal orientation, which was an intellectual learning based on the physical experience of festive and abundant eating. The Easter Bunny assured her that what she did was for her own benefit and not for the satisfaction of the adults. The holiday's great concentration on physical gratification guaranteed that she would continue to have her most primitive needs gratified no matter how she developed; she had by now seen for two years in a row that this was a tradition of the School for everyone.

The Easter baskets are full of candy and each contains two small toys. One of Rebecca's little toys was a game of jacks. A few days after Easter, her counselor invited her to play jacks. (As most of us remember, the equipment for this game consists of ten small metal stars called jacks and a small rubber ball. The player scatters the jacks in a limited area on the floor, then tosses the ball in the air, picks up one jack, and catches the ball after it has bounced one, and only one, time, all with one hand. The procedure is repeated until all of the jacks have been picked up. The jacks are then scattered again and picked up in the same manner two at a time, then three at a time, until finally all ten must be picked up at once.) Rebecca had attempted to play jacks on previous occasions with no success at all. While her approach this time was more willing, it was equally clumsy. However, this time, when her counselor explained her difficulty and how she might remedy it, she immediately put the verbal advice into physical effect and finished "ones" for the first time. Any mathematician who has finally found the solution to what has seemed an insoluble problem, any athlete who has finally mastered what has seemed an insurmountable height, and any of us who can remember our childhood, can understand the thrill of having "done my 'ones' for the first time." Nor did the IQ of 167 that enabled her to understand great complexities lessen the thrill, once the skill was within her grasp. Sitting on the floor with her legs crossed Indian style in front of her, bending her head, and bringing her arms close as though to hug herself, she said, "I'm pleased with myself"—a rare and beautiful statement from a child who felt herself so inadequate.

The particular difficulty that she had been having with jacks was that after she picked up the jack she would keep her fist closed over it so as to keep it from falling out of her hand; of course, she would then not be able to catch the ball. Her counselor simply explained that if she held her hand cupped, palm upward, the jack would be safe and she could still catch the ball. The crucial issue, of course, was that she could immediately use this intellectual knowledge to facilitate physical activity.

Playing ball became an important activity for Rebecca. She would spend much time playing not only jacks but also ball-bouncing games with the other girls, which were accompanied by recitation of a great variety of rhymes. These games involved an intellectual skill paralleling a physical skill. The importance of playing ball as a mastery in Rebecca's development as a whole person is perhaps best illustrated by the comparison of two incidents. A few months prior to learning to play ball-bouncing games, she had asked her counselor which was her right hand and which her left. She wanted to know because she knew that when she faced north, east would be on her right. This was typical of Rebecca, that she would know the distant, north and east, without having any notion of the immediate, right and left. She had no means available to find out which was which and, of course, did not know whether she was right- or left-handed. A few months after she learned to play with the ball she asked the same question for the same reason. This time she walked away before getting an answer and went through the motions of bouncing a ball. She came back, glowing with the answer to her question: "this" was her right hand because she knew for sure that she bounced the ball with her right hand. Her mastery of ball bouncing had provided the kinesthetically important sensation on which she could use her intelligence to solve the problem that concerned her. She could use her mind and body together to gain her own ends.

During the next months her desire and ability to master bodily activity blossomed. She had only begun to use utensils for eating, but she now decided that she wanted even to cut her meat by herself. Any form of washing was always extremely time-consuming for her, but she decided that she wanted to wash her hair herself. Since she could think about her body, she had begun to feel in control of it and wanted to assert her mastery. She explained that since she knew how her head felt she could tell better than her counselors when she was ready. She even decided to do her nails herself, believing that knowing how her own hands felt would compensate for her comparative lack of skill in filing and applying polish.

She learned how to ride a bicycle and to roller skate. In all of these activities it was surprisingly apparent that she was naturally extremely graceful. When her mind and body connected, she would learn a skill almost immediately. All of her bodily anxieties had by no means been resolved; at times the malfunctioning of her intellect in these efforts would appear alongside the useful functioning. If, for instance, she became anxious while skating, her movements would become caricatures of her usual graceful manner.

Rebecca would, of course, become discouraged at times and would need to be supported by the staff's delight, encouragement, and teaching. However, for each activity the initial incentive always came from within her. The activity that became most important to Rebecca was swimming, which involved significant body mastery and exposure, especially since it was water ballet that particularly interested her. That it involved both male and female instructors was probably also important. As with several of our activities that involve instructors with special skills, coordination between the skill expert (in this case the swimming instructor) and the person experts (in this case the counselors) is necessary. Our swimming period is supervised by a physical education teacher from the laboratory schools of the university, who at this time was a man. He gave lessons to Rebecca, both explaining and demonstrating the various strokes to her. She would watch and listen attentively and then, with her female counselor, practice what he had taught. So, both male and female instructors were involved in the encouragement and support of her physical movement and bodily exposure.

When Rebecca had reached a point of some security in the pleasure and advantage that she could derive from using mind and body together, she went on her first long visit home. The most importat emotional experience of the visit occurred to her not as an intellectual giant or a helpless infant, but as a more or less average young swimmer. Upon her return to the School it was evident that her swimming had much improved. She was able to pass the swimming test. She attributed her increased ability to the time she had spent at the local swimming pool with her stepsister, with whom for the first time she had been able to make friends, because of this common interest. Her ability to succeed in her home setting had great significance, because it was evidence of the contribution she had made to her own difficulties and, hence, of her ability to overcome them.

In addition to greater skill in swimming, Rebecca brought back with her a book on graphics that she had found in her local library. She announced that she was going to learn to read this book. At the time Rebecca was just beginning first-grade reading (she was ten), and this book, written on a young-adult level, was far beyond her reading ability. Her counselor told her that reading the book was out of the question. Rebecca was not discouraged, and, in order to prove herself capable, she agreed to try reading a paragraph, which her counselor had suggested to demonstrate how difficult it was. Very painstakingly, using all of the knowledge that she had so far acquired to figure out the words, she read the paragraph. The knowledge that had formerly led to such bizarre solutions, she could now really integrate with the material before her, to come exceedingly close to the right solution. Her counselor, surprised and delighted with her performance, was still concerned that the struggle would be too depleting of energy and too difficult to permit her to enjoy reading, so she offered to read the book to Rebecca so that she could satisfy her curiosity and be rewarded for her effort. However, it was of the utmost importance to Rebecca that she be the one to master this problem herself. She refused the offer and continued to insist on reading the book.

While the book was, according to accepted (and valid) teaching procedures, far too difficult to be a good choice, it offered what was worth the greatest difficulty: a solution to the basic mystery of reading. She could invest a great deal of energy in a book about how letters are formed and words are made, feeling that it was just the kind of knowledge that could lead to a mastery of reading; if she could find out how these words were made, she could master them.

Just as it was necessary that she have her teacher, the keeper of the intellectual, accompany her during her first physical mastery, so it was necessary that she have her counselor, the keeper of the physical, accompany her during her first purely intellectual mastery. The counselor's initial hesitation served the purpose of making it clear that the undertaking was truly Rebecca's desire. Every day she asked one of her counselors to read with her. At first she could do no more than one page a day, and often not even that. She was very insistent on two instructional methods and would become justifiably upset if they were not adhered to. Firstly, she did not want to be told what a word was, but rather how she could figure it out herself; in this way she was acquiring all the word-attack skills. (Since the counselors at the Orthogenic School are all involved in concurrent academic programs, it is not terribly unusual that they are familiar with educational principles; if not, they have access to appropriate resources.) She did not want to have the knowledge poured into her, nor did she want an incomprehensible fact presented to her. She wanted to master, understand, and be able to predict the sounds attached to these shapes and forms. Secondly, she was never satisfied with the mechanics of reading; she never left a sentence until she felt that she thoroughly understood its meaning. In this way she gained mastery and understanding of both the mechanical and the intellectual aspects of reading: of how the groups of letters sound and what they mean.

In the course of these reading sessions she at times began to revert to her old, unsuccessful, methods of decoding. This would invariably be a sign that she was angry or upset with her counselor and, for some reason, was unable to acknowledge it. Whenever she felt an injunction not to be aware of some feelings, her intellect could look at the words but had to protect itself from the danger of possible feelings. At these times her counselor would stop the reading and ask about the anger, thus directing her intellect to the problem and lifting the ban on seeing the anger. She could then go back to reading. She began her book in September and finished it in November. The following January she was reading a book from the Nancy Drew mystery series and articles on dance in the *New York Times*.

Three factors seemed to have led to Rebecca's ability to learn to read at this particular time. Firstly, it is likely that the impetus for her adamant insistence was that her counselor's "no" had made her so angry that she became determined to show her counselor that she was wrong. Secondly, she had finally the courage to approach reading without the feeling that she was going to fail. One of the sources of this courage was the feeling of someone beside her, for in order to have courage she had to have her counselor physically with her. It was not until she had almost completed the book that she would read by herself, although she no longer needed help. Thus she indicated the importance of the independence of her choice and of the support and approval of her counselors. It was the third element, however, that seemed the most important since the first two had been present at other times. She said that when she was on her visit she had swum a lot. She had first learned to swim at the School and had practiced more when she was at home; when she came back, she could pass the swimming test. She had found out with swimming that when she put in just a small amount of effort, she would get out a great amount of results. So, she thought, if this was true of swimming then perhaps it would be true of reading. And so it was that in four months she covered four years' progress in reading. The mastery of a physical activity had led directly to the mastery of an intellectual activity—the physical activity that she was able to master by turning her agile mind to her agile body.

EIGHT

Empathy
(The Heart of the Enterprise)

I began this book about education with a description of an external framework and a setting conducive to growth. I would like to end with a discussion of an internal foundation and an emotion essential to growth. Many modern practitioners believe empathy to be the basis of the psychoanalytic enterprise; I believe it should be an integral component of any human enterprise. I hope that an empathic attitude has pervaded this work, so that this last chapter need be only a brief exclamation point.

At one time when I was trying to organize my thoughts about the issue of empathy and children, I asked my son, who was nine years old, if he knew what empathy meant. He said, yeah, he thought it meant feeling like another person feels. I asked him how he knew that, since I hadn't seen the word on any of his fourth-grade vocabulary lists. It seemed that on a science fiction program he had seen a TV empathizer machine that went around making people feel the way the person on the TV felt. On further reflection, after consulting the psychoanalytic literature, colleagues, and the Oxford dictionary, I realized that while my son's might be a popular definition, it is not what I or any of my colleagues in either mental health or teaching mean by empathy. The difference is that the empathy that is vital in dealing effectively with other human beings takes an active effort on the part of one person, on behalf of another. What the so-called empathizer machine produced was an automatic response. For example, the empathizer machine would make a teacher, on observing an anxious and insecure student, also feel anxious and insecure.

This reaction happens frequently enough in real life, and we can frequently enough see the unfortunate results. One young woman was preparing to leave the School and considering taking a high school equivalency exam. She was extraordinarily anxious about it. Her teacher became anxious with her and agreed that she should not take it. Further discussion with other members of the staff led to the conclusion that, though the young woman might not be entirely prepared for the test, her anxiety was typical of her approach to any new challenge in life and, therefore, what she needed was encouragement to try for success, and preparation to deal with possible failure. She passed the test. This young woman had a mother who had been deeply sensitive to her as a small child and would respond to her distress with similar distress. Her mother's response led to more distress on the part of the child, because seeing her mother as anxious as she would confirm her sad view of the world. Doctors often see similar reactions and at times wisely prefer to have mothers leave the examining room. In anticipation of her return to life with or near her family, we tried to help this young woman be aware of her mother's propensity to become worried with her. She was already very much aware of her own tendency to become exceedingly anxious when she was about to undertake a new responsibility and she realized that she would have to reassure her mother, so that her mother's reaction to her anxiety would not impede her own mastery of it and her forward progression.

A truly empathic teacher, on observing an anxious student, might have revived the emotional memories of being an anxious and insecure student. Recognizing that the anxiety has been stimulated, not by being in the problematic situation but by the student's being there, the teacher could make use of the reaction to understand better the student's anxiety. The teacher's new understanding could lead to the creation of conditions that would likely alleviate the anxiety and facilitate the progress of learning. The importance of the distinction being made is immediately apparent when we think of the problem of contagion. When a child is angry, another child seeing the anger might become angry also. This reaction is neither what we call empathy nor what we want to happen. The beginning of empathy is when seeing a child angry leads to a thoughtful recognition of the anger and consideration of its sources: "Why might I be angry in that place?" In order to really answer that question one has to reexperience in a small dose the emotion (anger, in this case) that one has felt in the past. Full empathy is the use of the understanding thus gained to relieve the stress of the other person.

Since we consider empathy to be of great value, we spend a great deal of time and energy developing empathic avenues for our staff, as discussed in earlier chapters. We find many times that though the desire to be empathic exists (it would be unusual for anyone coming to work at an institution such as the Orthogenic School not to have such a desire), as does the skill, there are certain feelings and anxieties that interfere. Perhaps most obvious is simple anger at being mistreated. As one staff member quoted earlier put it, "It's easy enough to be understanding when a kid is lying on his bed crying about how bad he feels. It's a lot harder when he's attacking you."

A number of anxieties seem typical in preventing people from feeling empathic. One very frequent anxiety is related to recognizing in oneself a similarity to someone whom one considers "strange." Freud referred to this anxiety when he spoke against referring to a sexually different way of acting as a perversion, because, he said, when something is viewed as perverse, it is more difficult for people to empathize with it. Often when I have strongly denied to a student that a friend's behavior or feeling is aberrant, the student will reveal having engaged in similar behavior or having had similar feelings. Many a child has revealed an attachment to a stuffed animal or a piece of material after we have insisted that having infantile desires does not make a person a "baby." Recently a young man was telling me about a high school friend who considered herself a lesbian. She had told him that when she was younger she had always had crushes on other girls rather than on boys and that she considered this an early sign of lesbian tendencies. When I said that attractions to members of the same sex were not unusual for anyone, he recalled that he had had fascinations with other boys. Since his identity was strongly heterosexual, he had not been able to think of his experience empathically with hers, if it might identify him as a homosexual. When my reassurance had allayed this anxiety, he could think of his similar experience.

The fear of being entirely like the person with whom one

shares some feelings is often a major source of difficulty in classrooms, when a particular child is seen as ugly, stupid, or strange. Other children are afraid of understanding how that child feels, afraid of recognizing that there might be any similarity between them, because that would mean that they, too, are ugly, stupid, or strange. Staff who work with very disturbed people also have such reactions. When they see something in the disturbed one that is similar to themselves, they fear it means they, too, are seriously disturbed. A very empathic, talented teacher related her experience in a psychiatric hospital. When she talked to other staff members about herself experiencing a feeling one of the patients had expressed, they acted somewhat horrified that she would consider herself to be like a psychotic person.

This issue is human and understandable, but provides a great interference with the use of one of the most valuable tools in our work. In order to understand another most thoroughly, we have to understand the other's emotion in ourselves. Unless we can have the feeling "There but for the grace of God go I," we are not able to have the kind of alliance that is essential to any common enterprise involving emotional interaction, be it therapy or learning.

Another frequent anxiety that interferes with the very beginning of empathy is that some terrible feelings might be stirred up. When I see someone acting miserable, if I really try to feel as that person, then I am going to experience some painful feelings; I am going to be reminded of situations that I do not want to remember, because it will hurt to do so. This is often the reason that staff members find themselves avoiding certain students, or avoiding thinking about certain students. These students are often those with whom we have the most significant issues in common and, therefore, with whom we have the greatest potential to be empathic.

Children similarly try to avoid the arousal of painful feelings. We find that frequently our children have some signal of empathic response which leads them to engage in a variety of maneuvers to avoid having to suffer the extreme discomfort it begins to arouse. Aggressive children, upon seeing someone very sad or anxious, will initiate some very stimulating activity—joking, horseplay—to "drown out" the sadness or anxiety. Very often children who get into trouble together have very similar emotional memories; many stimuli evoke very similar responses in them. Seeing each other in emotionally difficult situations elicits empathic responses, the painfulness of which they join forces to avoid. Since frequently their unity is in socially disapproved behavior, we tend to see their united front as against adults, rather than as against experiencing their own misery.

In general, the kind of anxieties that may stand in the way of empathic response to disturbed children are neither unusual nor unhealthy. It is often useful in a staff member's personal development to rework some issues that are stirred up in contact with disturbed youngsters, but it is seldom absolutely necessary for living a fruitful life. In order to be empathic with an aggressive child, one has to be in touch with one's own aggressive feelings; with a depressed child, one has to be familiar with one's own depressiveness. Many staff members have found this familiarity to be helpful in gaining mastery over their inner lives and in gaining greater equanimity and security. But for many others, the rewards are not worth the pain. It is both a benefit and a hazard of our work that in order to be empathic, one often has to confront difficult, conflictual issues in oneself that one might otherwise live happily without having met. In order to understand and master the issues that are aroused in this work and interfere with empathy, staff members often decide to go into psychotherapy. Psychoanalysis or other forms of psychoanalytic psychotherapy can be very helpful in enabling a staff member to become more aware of unintegrated emotions and thereby to be able to be more empathic with psychically disintegrated students.

In many instances a staff member, despite experiencing anger at being attacked, and despite the anxieties discussed, is able to respond empathically. I have earlier referred to the staff member who described how a boy would call her "nigger" when he became frustrated building with plastic Lego blocks. She at first reacted by insisting that he not talk that way to her and withdrew; he would become more abusive, and the situation would deteriorate more. Finally, on one such occasion she heard him saying, "I can't learn, I can't ever do this." She suddenly realized that it was out of his feeling of being defeat-

144

CHAPTER EIGHT

ed that he was saying just the thing that would arouse her associations of being defeated. She then could begin to use her feelings as an empathic response, as an avenue to understanding and helpful activity, rather than to reactivity and withdrawal. She told him that he could learn, that she would sit with him and help him and not let either of them be defeated, whereupon they had a series of successful learning experiences around the building blocks.

How was she able to regain an empathic stance? The staff needs a great deal of mutual support in order to be empathic in the face of quite natural self-protective devices. The first support is in strongly held mores that the students, no matter how aberrant their behavior, can be understood, and in the same terms that we understand ourselves. This conviction should not be construed to imply that the staff at all times can be expected to be able to be empathic. However, it permits a staff member to return to an empathic stance after being attacked or barraged by chaotic emotions and having reacted perhaps negatively. These mores allow a staff member to become angry at or hurt by a student's behavior and still remain on the student's side, by afterwards understanding the source of the student's actions, rather than concluding that the student is bad or crazy.

Staff members at the same time need a great deal of mutual support in accepting the naturalness of their own negative reactions. In discussions of the incident just described, it was important for other staff members to try to help the counselor, both in understanding the actions of the youngster and in sympathizing with her natural anger at being called "nigger." Both kinds of support are needed. If the only support given is for the staff member's hurt at being subjected to assault, the staff is likely to be "down" on the student. However, if the only support given is for the understanding of the student, then the staff is likely to be "down" on the staff member who is not able to be empathic. All staff groups that I have known have been susceptible to erring in both directions.

Since access to our own feelings is in our view only the beginning of empathy, we also have to devote much time and energy to understanding how to utilize these feelings in the best interest of our students. Quite often, when one is motivated to try to put onself in the skin of another and is able to find an experience similar enough to recall a similar emotion, one then so well knows what to do that doing it is automatic, and it is impossible even to recapture the critical acts. In the case of the boy who tore his clothes, once the counselor had access to her own empathic reaction and could sort it out to be able to separate the aspects that belonged to her own particular psychology, she could behave in such a way as to alleviate the boy's need to tear his clothes. In dealing with the epidemic of swearing at the nursery school and day-care center, we asked each teacher to express her view in regard to the swearing. One of the most articulate of the teachers said that she actually enjoyed the freedom the children had to do something that she would never have been able to do as a child. In explicating her feeling she was able to see that her enjoyment was not good for what she really thought best for the child. In the few days following the teachers' meeting to discuss the issue, though no course of action had been decided upon, the swearing almost entirely vanished. Once the teachers had clarified their feelings, it appeared that they could combine their initial empathic reactions with the skills they had to convey to their charges that swearing was not a good idea.

It does not always work this way. A teacher told me that she was sure she just could not be empathic with Sue. She said that ever since she had started working with Sue, people had told her that she should think about how would she feel if she held herself in that position (and she mimicked the position in which the girl often held herself). She said that she knew it was utter misery, but knowing that did not help her to know what to do when she saw the girl in that way expressing her misery. "I know whenever I leave, like for staff meeting [a time when Sue typically held herself in the position], what she feels is desertion, utter desertion. And people say that I should think about what I would have liked someone to do for me, but what can you do for a person in that situation, short of just staying." It was clear from the way she said it that the teacher was being reminded of a real desertion in her own past. Without having to go into the details of her own experience, it was possible to point out to the teacher that, while the feeling that the empathy evoked was accurate to the feeling of misery of the girl, the present situation of the girl was not the same as the situation that had evoked the teacher's desperate feeling in the past. That is, the teacher had felt that miserable herself when she was really significantly deserted. The girl, while feeling desperate, was not in reality being deserted. Though the teacher was leaving, she would be back in a short time. Once the teacher had made the distinction for herself, she could make the distinction for the girl. She could express sympathy for the girl's real pain and at the same time clarify the real situation. I believe that our avenue for discovering what to do is careful examination and reexamination of the details of the situation and of student's reactions, with our minds and with our hearts.

We make no particular effort to teach empathy to the children at the Orthogenic School. They do not have, until they are close to leaving us, enough emotional energy to be able to invest that much in another's welfare, nor have they mastery enough of their past emotional experiences. However, we do a number of things that I believe foster the development of empathy in them, not the least of which is to provide, we hope, models for them. It is quite striking that, around issues that they are not afraid to think about, issues about which they feel that they have received sufficient gratification and a pretty good understanding, they are able to act in ways reflecting empathy.

This occurred, for example, when we took in a school-phobic teenager. She came on a Friday afternoon, spent a few minutes in class, and then on Monday morning would not get out of bed. After being enticed out of bed with some food served to her by hand, she still refused to go to class. So we had the class go to her. They all went over to her dormitory and did their work there. The class members, including two very aggressive, acting-out boys, were utterly well-behaved and cooperative. They talked with her about the difficulties of being in a new, strange place and about other things that might make her uncomfortable. These very disturbed children were able to do this because they had before her coming discussed their feelings about the difficulties of putting up with the disruption of a new kid and had reminisced about how they had felt and had been catered to when they were new.

They were thus prepared and able to easily put themselves in her place, to remember having had a similar emotion, to feel how it felt, and since it had been mastered well, to know how to be helpful to her. The new girl went to class that afternoon and continued to go to class thereafter. She would not have been able to do so if the other children had only remembered how it felt to be new. It was their empathic effort to make her feel better that enabled her to join them.

I very strongly believe that our purpose in teaching our children is to help them to be able to master their inner and outer lives, so that they can be the people they want to be and achieve the goals they want to achieve. I must confess that when they act as they did toward the frightened new girl (as they often do), I am pleased and proud. It confirms my idea that a mind well nurtured can learn the lessons of both the intellectual and emotional worlds.

NOTES

Introduction

1. Bruno Bettelheim, *Love is Not Enough* (New York: The Free Press, 1950).
2. Bruno Bettelheim, *Truants from Life* (Glencoe, Ill.: The Free Press, 1955).
3. Bruno Bettelheim, *The Empty Fortress* (New York: The Free Press, 1967).
4. Bruno Bettelheim, *A Home for the Heart* (New York: Alfred A. Knopf, 1974).
5. The theoretical organization of my thinking has been especially influenced by David Rapaport, "The Structure of Psycho-analytic Theory," in Sigmund Koch, ed., *Psychology: A Study of a Science*, vol. 3 (New York: McGraw-Hill, 1959), 55–183; and Merton M. Gill, ed. *The Collected Papers of David Rapaport* (New York: Basic Books, 1967).

Chapter One

1. My theoretical notions have, of course, been digested over many years from much material. The works that have best, concisely summarized the theory for me are Sigmund Freud, *An Outline of Psychoanalysis* (New York: W. W. Norton & Co., 1949); and Charles Brenner, *An Elementary Textbook of Psychoanalysis* (New York: International Universities Press, 1955).
2. Maria Montessori, *The Montessori Method* (Cambridge, Mass.: Robert Bentley, 1964).
3. This summary also draws especially from Erik Erikson, *Childhood and Society* (New York: W. W. Norton & Co., 1950); and Anna Freud, *Normality and Pathology in Childhood* (New York: International Universities Press, 1965).

Chapter Three

1. Montessori, *The Montessori Method*.
2. Erikson, *Childhood and Society*, 247–74.

NOTES

Chapter Four

1. The summary of Erikson's stages is based on my understanding of Erikson, *Childhood and Society*, 247–74; and Erik Erikson, "Identity and the Lifecycle," *Psychological Issues* 1, no. 1 (1959).

2. Sylvia Ashton-Warner, *Teacher* (New York: Simon & Shuster, 1963).

Chapter Five

1. Gregory Bateson, D. D. Jackson, J. Haley, and J. Weakland, "Toward a Theory of Schophrenia," *Behavioral Science* 1 (1956).

Chapter Six

1. Ashton-Warner, *Teacher*.

2. David Rapaport, "The Theory of Attention Cathexis," in *The Collected Papers of David Rapaport*, 778–94.

3. My understanding of Anna Freud's ideas is based, of course, on more than one work. That which is particularly pertinent is *Normality and Pathology in Childhood*.

4. Lili Peller, "Libidinal Phases, Ego Development and Play," in *The Psychoanalytic Study of the Child*, vol. 9, ed. Albert J. Solnit and Peter B. Neubauer (New York: International Universities Press, 1954), 178–98.

5. Erikson, *Childhood and Society*.

6. Freud, *Normality and Pathology in Childhood*, 62–68.

7. Carolyn Haywood, *Little Eddie* (New York: William Morrow & Co., 1947). This is one of many similar books by this author.

8. Peller, "Libidinal Phases."

9. Peller, "Libidinal Phases," 190–91.

10. The analysis of this class was more fully presented in two papers coauthored by the teacher of the class, who developed the curriculum in consultation with me, recorded the course of action, and did much of the analysis of the results: Ruth Andrea Levinson and Jacquelyn Sanders, "Student Engagement in Learning: A Psychoanalytic Perspective in the Development of Curricula" (paper delivered at the Annual Meeting of the American Educational Research Association, San Francisco, April, 1986); and Ruth Andrea Levinson and Jacquelyn Sanders, "An Educational Curriculum and the Psychological Needs of the Student: A Case Study of Interactions" (paper delivered at the Annual Meeting of the American Orthopsychiatric Association, Chicago, April, 1986).

$INDEX$

Ability grouping, reactions to, 89
Abstraction, value of to children, 121
Abused children, reaction of to punishment, 50–51
Acceptance: support for attitude of, 27; difficulty in acquiring attitude of, 26; and attention cathexis 113
Adaptation, ego as organ of, 105
Adjustment, initial, to Orthogenic School, 118
Admission: criteria for, 4; first interview for, 116
Adolescence, in Erikson's framework, 71
Allowance: purpose of, 125; restriction of as punishment, 53
Anal stage, 68
Anal sublimations, examples of, 106–7
Anger: and empathy, 140; dealing with reaction of, 87
Animal study curriculum, 109–10
Animals, stuffed: significance of, 124–25; tradition of, 124–25
Anorexic girl, example of interaction with, 67
Anxiety: and attention cathexis, 102; dealing with in the curriculum 93; about injury in physical education, 70; interference with empathy, 141–43; in latency, 107; and learning, 75, 94, 102; effect on of mode of presentation, 112–13
Arts, time of class, 60
Ashton-Warner, Sylvia, 73, 100

Associate Director, responsibility of, 13–14
Attention-cathexis, 100–103
Attitude, therapeutic, 21; of acceptance, 26, 27; toward autistic children, 22; toward bizarre behavior, 120; children observing staff's, toward other children, 120; psychoanalytic, 22; toward psychotic children, 22
Authority, 13–14, 15
Autistic child, example of behavior of, 24
Autistic children: therapeutic attitude toward, 22; and eye contact, 23–24
Autonomy vs. shame and doubt: 68; application of to curriculum, 68–69
Average expectable environment, 63–65
Aversive measures: as ego support, 47; alleviating guilt, 47; need for, 35–36. See also Punishment

Barnacle, response to in curriculum, 113
Bateson, Gregory, 92–93
Bedtime, preparation for, 124
Beginning of school day, 59–60
Bettelheim, Bruno, 3, 11, 13; books by, xiv
Biology: as anxiety-arousing subject matter, 75–76, 93–94; as cathected subject matter, 75; example of psychological problem, 93

154

Initiative vs. guilt (continued)
Orthogenic School curriculum,
69–70
Insects, class reaction to, 93
Insults, reaction to and
understanding of, 85

"Jacks," 132

Kitchen staff, importance of, 16

Latency, 70; in relationship to
beginning reading, 70
Libidinal energy, 68
Literature, as example of
appropriate curriculum, 95
Living room, description of, 11

Mammary glands, response to in
curriculum, 112
Masochistic fantasies, and hitting,
51
Math: attitudes toward, 88; time of
class, 60
Maturation, 105
Meetings, format of: with
Orthogenic School teachers, 83;
with nursery school teachers in
training, 83–85
Mental apparatus, structure of, 17
Milieu therapy, author's
interpretation of, 21
Mirror, importance of, 129–31
Montessori, Maria, 10, 36
Mores, in support of empathy, 144
Motivation, for work at Orthogenic
School, 81
Motive-relevant curriculum,
example of, 110
Motives, and attention cathexis, 103
Mutuality, importance in
development of control, 45

Name-calling, reaction to, 83–85
Needs, consideration of child's in
planning of curriculum, 96
Night, dealing with a problem of,
31, 119

Night counselor, 119
Nuisance, response to topic of, in
curriculum, 113
Nursery school, format of seminar
at, 83
Nursing, response to topic of, in
curriculum, 112
Nurturance: need for in
adolescence, 67; response to topic
of, in curriculum, 111

Oedipal conflict, in regard to
learning to read, 104
One-look words, 73
Oral stage, 17
Orderliness, in development of
discipline, 36–37
Organization, temporal: in class, 58;
in development of discipline, 37
Orientation in time, development
of, 131
Orientation to new environment,
118
Orthogenic School, the Sonia
Shankman, of the University of
Chicago: books about, xiv;
description of, 10; history of, xi;
identification, 2; work of, 19

Parental figures, as subject matter,
105
Peer group, importance of in
latency, 107; importance of in
stage of identity vs. role
diffusion, 71
Peller, Lili, 101, 106
Phallic stage, 69
Physical education: anxiety about
injury in, 70; competitive aspects
of, 70; example of value, 108;
importance, 60; in relationship to
initiative vs. guilt, 70
Physical education teacher,
importance of, 15
Physical environment, essential
components of, 7

Play: in relationship to beginning reading, 106; value of in treatment, 122
Primary process, danger in, 28
Primitive issues in curriculum, 109
Privacy, 7
Privileges, withdrawal of, as punishment, 52–53
Psychic/emotional curriculum, 62–72
Psychic energy, 17
Psychic striving, 101
Psychoanalysis: as avenue to empathy, 143; value of staff's in work, 33
Psychoanalytically oriented milieu therapy, definition of, 67
Psychoanalytic attitude, components of, 22
Psychoanalytic consultants, 14
Psychoanalytic ego psychology, 16
Psychological Problems in the Classroom, graduate course, 83
Psychologist, characteristics and responsibilities of, 14
Psychotherapy as avenue to empathy, 143
Psychotic children, therapeutic attitude toward, 22, 24–25
Psychotropic medication, use of, 3
Punishment: as deterrent, 48; as ego support, 47; to alleviate guilt, 47; as clear message about standards, 46; need for, 35–36; as protection to others, 49; modes of 50–54

Questioning, as didactic technique, 92–93

Rapaport, David, xv, 100, 102, 103
Reading: high school, as example of psychological consideration, 96; time of class, 60
Reality testing, 17
Restitutive activity: in development of discipline, 45; as punishment, 51–52

Restriction on activities as punishment, 53
Robinson Crusoe, appeal of, 106
Routines, and interference with understanding, 87
Rules: importance in latency, 107; at Orthogenic school, 39

Safety, importance of, 7, 70
School phobic child: needs of, 61; example of dealing with, 146–47
Science laboratory course, example of value of, 108
Self-control, 21, 36–42
Self-knowledge, value of, 29–30, 88
Separation from parents, 116–17
Session rooms, 10
Sessions at the School, purpose of, 15
Severely disturbed students, impact of on other students, 120
Sex, response to topic of, in curriculum, 111
Social anthropology, as class for stage of identity vs. role diffusion, 71–72
Social studies, example of discussion group, 93
Social worker, characteristics and responsibilities of, 14
Speed, unit on, as example of appropriate nursery school curriculum, 97
Sperm-conducting organ, response to topic of, in curriculum, 112
Stress, in relationship to development of discipline, 41
Structural development, psychic, 105
Structuralization, 105
Structure and function, response to, in biology curriculum, 112
Students: diagnoses, xiii; follow-up, xiii; general description, 5–6; nature of, 2
Suckling to rational eating (developmental line), 105